TABLE OF CONTENTS

About the Authors 2

Preface 3

Introduction 4

WHITE LESIONS 15

RED LESIONS 35

ULCERATED LESIONS 51

BLISTERING / SLOUGHING LESIONS 73

PIGMENTED LESIONS 87

PAPILLARY LESIONS 99

SOFT TISSUE ENLARGEMENTS 109

DRUG SECTION

    Alphabetical Listing of Drugs Commonly Used in the Treatment of
        Oral Soft Tissue Diseases 133

    Example Prescriptions 147

SPECIAL TOPICS

    Management of Patients Undergoing Cancer Therapy 156
        Oral Lesions in Cancer Treatment 157
    Dry Mouth (Xerostomia) 159
        Artificial Saliva Products 159
        Other Dry Mouth Products 159
        Cholinergic Salivary Stimulants (Rx only) 160
    Fluorides 161
        Prescription Only Products 161
        Over-the-Counter Products 161
    Preprocedural Antibiotics in Dental Patients 162
    HIV Infection and AIDS 166
        Natural History of HIV Infection / Oral Manifestations 166
        CD4+ Lymphocyte Count and Percentage as Related to the Risk of
            Opportunistic Infection 166
        Oral Lesions Commonly Seen in HIV / AIDS 166
    Normal Blood Values 167
    Suggested Readings 168

ANATOMIC SITE INDEX 173

ALPHABETICAL INDEX 179

ABOUT THE AUTHORS

J. Robert Newland, DDS, MS

After more than 20 years as a dental educator, Dr Newland recently left academic dentistry to devote himself to his private practice in Houston, Texas. Before leaving academic dentistry, Dr Newland served in both faculty and administrative positions at the University of Texas Health Science Center at Houston, Dental Branch, including Chair of the Department of Diagnostic Sciences and Associate Dean for Student Affairs. Dr Newland graduated from the University of Texas in 1966 and received a Doctor of Dental Surgery Degree from the University of Texas Health Science Center at Houston, Dental Branch in 1970. He completed an Advanced Education Program in Oral Pathology at the University of Texas Health Science Center at Houston, Dental Branch and received a Master of Science Degree in Oral Pathology in 1978. Dr Newland also completed a fellowship in Oral Pathology at the MD Anderson Cancer Center. He has written more than 100 scientific publications on a variety of topics related to his specialty, including benign and malignant oral tumors, oral manifestations of HIV infection and AIDS, oral manifestations of systemic diseases, and the diagnosis and treatment of oral soft tissue diseases. Dr Newland has presented more than 100 continuing education seminars to dental and medical healthcare providers. He has maintained an active private practice for more than 18 years where he manages patients with a wide range of oral diseases.

Timothy F. Meiller, DDS, PhD

Dr Meiller is Professor of Diagnostic Sciences and Pathology at the Baltimore College of Dental Surgery and Professor of Oncology in the Program of Oncology at the Greenebaum Cancer Center, University of Maryland Baltimore. He has held his position in Diagnostic Sciences at the Dental School for 26 years and serves as an attending faculty at the Greenebaum Cancer Center. Dr Meiller is a Diplomate of the American Board of Oral Medicine and a graduate of Johns Hopkins University and the University of Maryland Dental and Graduate Schools, holding a DDS and a PhD in Immunology/Virology. He has over 200 publications to his credit, maintains an active general dental practice, and is a consultant to the National Institutes of Health. He is currently engaged in ongoing investigations into cellular immune dysfunction in oral diseases associated with AIDS, in cancer patients, and in other medically-compromised patients.

Richard L. Wynn, BSPharm, PhD

Richard L. Wynn, PhD, is Professor of Pharmacology at the Baltimore College of Dental Surgery, Dental School, University of Maryland Baltimore. Dr Wynn has served as a dental educator, researcher, and teacher of dental pharmacology and dental hygiene pharmacology for his entire professional career. He holds a BS (pharmacy; registered pharmacist, Maryland), an MS (physiology) and a PhD (pharmacology) from the University of Maryland. Dr Wynn chaired the Department of Pharmacology at the University of Maryland Dental School from 1980 to 1995. Previously, he chaired the Department of Oral Biology at the University of Kentucky College of Dentistry. Dr Wynn has to his credit over 300 publications including original research articles, textbooks, textbook chapters, monographs, and articles in continuing education journals. He has given over 500 continuing education seminars to dental professionals in the U.S., Canada, and Europe. Dr Wynn has been a consultant to the drug industry for 22 years and his research laboratories have contributed to the development of new analgesics and anesthetics. He is a consultant to the U.S. Pharmacopeia, Dental Drugs and Products section, the Academy of General Dentistry, the American Dental Association, and a former consultant to the Council on Dental Education, Commission on Accreditation. He is a featured columnist and his drug review articles, entitled *Pharmacology Today*, appear in each issue of *General Dentistry*, a journal published by the Academy. One of his primary interests continues to be keeping dental professionals informed on all aspects of drug use in dental practice.

Harold L. Crossley, DDS, PhD

Dr Crossley is Professor Emeritus at the Baltimore College of Dental Surgery, Dental School, University of Maryland Baltimore. A native of Rhode Island, he received a Bachelor of Science degree in Pharmacy from the University of Rhode Island in 1964. He later was awarded the Master of Science (1970) and Doctorate degrees (1972) in the area of Pharmacology. The University of Maryland Dental School in Baltimore awarded Dr Crossley the DDS degree in 1980. He is the Director of Conjoint Sciences and Preclinical Studies at the School of Dentistry and maintains an intramural part-time private dental practice. Dr Crossley has coauthored a number of articles dealing with law enforcement on both a local and federal level. This liaison with law enforcement agencies keeps him well-acquainted with the "drug culture." He has been appointed to the Governor's Commission on Prescription Drug Abuse and the Maryland State Dental Association's Well-Being Committee. Drawing on this unique background, Dr Crossley has become nationally and internationally recognized as an expert on street drugs and chemical dependency, as well as the clinical pharmacology of dental drugs.

PREFACE

Some oral soft tissue diseases exhibit distinctive clinical features and only require visual recognition to establish an accurate diagnosis. Others share common clinical features and present a diagnostic challenge even for the most experienced clinician. Recognizing the clinical features most helpful in differentiating one lesion from another is an essential part of the diagnostic process. We have prepared *Diagnosis and Management of Oral Soft Tissue Diseases: A Reference Manual for Dental Practitioners* to address this challenge by presenting the information necessary to diagnose and manage oral soft tissue diseases in a format that suits the needs of the busy dental practitioner.

The components of the diagnostic process are presented in the introductory section of the manual. Each of the next seven sections is devoted to a specific diagnostic category (white lesions, red lesions, ulcerated lesions, blistering/sloughing lesions, pigmented lesions, papillary lesions, and soft tissue enlargements). We have not attempted to include all the lesions that might conceivably fit a specific diagnostic category. Rather, we have focused on lesions that 1) are likely to be encountered in a general dental practice, 2) represent a specific differential diagnostic challenge, 3) may be associated with potentially life-threatening disease, or 4) may pose an occupational risk to members of the dental team. Each of the lesions included in a diagnostic category is illustrated with one or more high quality, full-color photographs intended to depict typical clinical features. Concise drug monographs and sample prescriptions comprise the next section of the manual, and the final section contains information related to special topics such as the treatment of oral mucosal lesions associated with cancer chemotherapy and chronic dry mouth.

We do not want this manual to languish on your bookshelf. We hope that you will find it so useful that it will be kept at chair-side where it can assist you with the diagnosis and management of your patients with oral soft tissue diseases.

J. Robert Newland

Timothy F. Meiller

Richard L. Wynn

Harold L. Crossley

INTRODUCTION

The soft tissues of the oral cavity are the site of a variety of diseases. Some of these diseases exhibit distinctive clinical features which enable the clinician to make a diagnosis with confidence. Others share common features making the diagnosis more difficult. The diagnosis of many oral soft tissue diseases can be a challenge even for the experienced clinician.

The purpose of this visually-cued manual is to assist you in recognizing the most diagnostic clinical features of oral soft tissue diseases. This image-driven process correlates the clinical presentation of each lesion with underlying pathologic changes. These visual cues coupled with patient history enable you to begin the diagnostic process.

The first section of this manual includes information about the diagnostic process (obtaining a history, examining the patient, recording historical and clinical data, establishing a differential diagnosis), and selecting appropriate diagnostic procedures (eg, biopsy, brush biopsy, and exfoliative cytology). Once a diagnosis is made, it is important for you to decide if it is appropriate to treat the lesion yourself, or to refer the patient for treatment. It is also necessary to assess results of treatment and re-evaluate the patient at appropriate intervals.

The body of the manual is divided into seven sections, each representing a specific diagnostic category. These diagnostic categories include:

- White Lesions
- Red Lesions
- Ulcerated Lesions
- Blistering / Sloughing Lesions
- Pigmented Lesions
- Papillary Lesions
- Soft Tissue Enlargements

On the pages that follow, each tab represents the general diagnostic category of the lesions included. It should be remembered that these diagnostic categories are somewhat arbitrary and that there may be overlap between them. A particular lesion is included in a category based on its most common clinical presentation.

For each disease included in a diagnostic category, the following information is presented:

- Most common name for the lesion
- Synonyms for the lesion including alternative naming schemes that may have historical importance (thus facilitating communication among clinicians)
- Brief discussion of the etiology
- One or more images of a typical lesion with a description of the clinical features emphasizing those of greatest diagnostic value (the most common clinical manifestations, as well as clinical variations are presented)

- Other useful clinical information, including symptoms and epidemiologic data
- Differential diagnosis
- Appropriate diagnostic steps
- Recommended treatment
- Follow-up, if appropriate
- Clinical significance (eg, could the lesion indicate the presence of a serious systemic disease, be potentially life-threatening, or represent a hazard to the clinician?)

The next section of this manual presents alphabetical arranged and cross-referenced monographs of drug mentioned in the treatment sections of each disease. In the section you will find example prescriptions for common medications useful in the management of the oral medicine conditions. The "Special Topics" section contains valuable information about the management of oral lesions patients receiving cancer therapy, management of oral lesions associated with chronic dry mouth, fluoride supplements, preprocedural antibiotics in dental patients, HIV infection and AIDS, and normal blood values. There is also a suggested reading list for those who want to learn more about the various topics presented.

THE DIAGNOSTIC PROCESS

The first step in the diagnostic process is to have the patient complete a health questionnaire. The health questionnaire should provide information that will enable you assess the patient's......

- overall health status (general health)
- disease history (serious illnesses, hospitalizations surgical procedures)
- current medications (over-the-counter and prescription)
- allergies (drugs, foods, other)
- social history (tobacco, alcohol, and/or recreation drug exposure)
- family history (health status of family members)

The health questionnaire should also contain a place for the patient to describe his/her chief complaint.

Next, you should interview the patient to obtain a complete history. Information provided by the patient in the health questionnaire will serve as a guide for the interview. The patient history should include the following:

- **Chief Complaint**

  If the patient is aware of the lesion, a description of it in the patient's own words.

- **History of Present Illness**

  Onset of the lesion - how long has the lesion been present? In general, lesions which persist for more than a few weeks are of greater concern.

Clinical course of the lesion - has the lesion increased in size, decreased in size, fluctuated in size, or remained stable?

Symptoms of the lesion - is the lesion painful? In the absence of pain, the patient may not be aware of the lesion. This is significant because oral cancers are often initially painless.

- **Relevant Medical History**

 Is there anything in the patient's medical history that might contribute to the diagnosis?

 Is the patient taking any medications that could be involved in the oral changes?

- **Relevant Dental History**

 Is there anything in the patient's dental history that might contribute to the diagnosis (eg, does the patient wear a prostheses, is there a history of trauma)?

All information obtained during the patient interview should be carefully recorded.

At the completion of the patient interview, a complete examination of the structures of the head and neck (extraoral examination) and oral cavity (intraoral examination) should be performed.

GENERAL PRINCIPLES OF EXTRAORAL AND INTRAORAL EXAMINATIONS

- A good light source is essential for adequate visual examination.

- Use a systematic approach for the examination.

- You must be familiar with the normal structures underlying the tissues you are palpating.

- You must know the normal appearance (normal anatomic variation) of the tissues you are inspecting in order to assess abnormalities.

- Obtain data by palpation and visual inspection.

- For bilateral structures, compare the appearance of one side with the other.

- For oral soft tissues supported by bone (attached gingiva and mucosa of the hard palate), palpate by compressing the tissues against the bone.

- For tissues not supported by bone, palpate between the fingers.

- Carefully record the findings.

COMPONENTS OF THE EXTRAORAL EXAMINATION

Examination of the Head

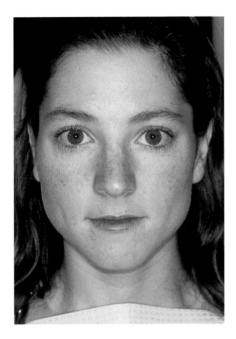

- Evaluate facial symmetry - are any areas of facial swelling present?

- Inspect the skin - what is the texture of the skin? Are any lesions present?

- Inspect the eyes - is there any evidence of conjunctival inflammation or other lesions?

- Evaluate eye movements - are the eye movements normal?

- Inspect the nose - are there any asymmetries? Is there any discharge?

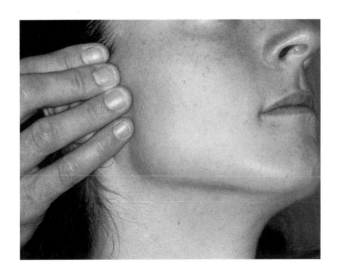

- Palpate the temporomandibular joints - using light pressure, place your fingers just anterior to the tragus. Instruct the patient to slowly open, close, and move the mandible from one side to the other.

INTRODUCTION *(Continued)*

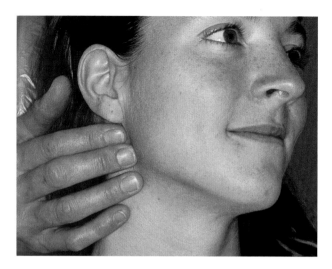

- Palpate the parotid salivary glands - using light pressure, place your fingers at the angles of the mandible over the parotid glands. Normal parotid glands are usually not palpable.

Examination of the Neck

Note: Palpation of the structures of the neck can be performed most efficiently when the clinician stands behind the patient.

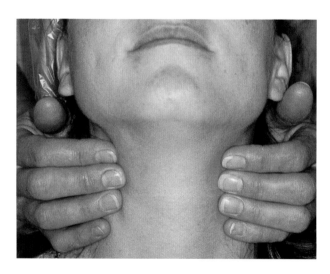

- Palpate the sternocleidomastoid muscle, the midline structures of the neck, and the cervicle lymph nodes.

Note: Enlarged lymph nodes can result from an infectious/inflammatory process or a malignant neoplasm (primary or metastatic). The clinical characteristics of the enlarged lymph node can help differentiate between the two.

Lymph nodes enlarged because of an infectious/inflammatory process are generally:

- Soft to palpation
- Freely movable
- Painful

Lymph nodes enlarged because of a primary or maligna neoplasm are generally:

- Firm to palpation
- Fixed to adjacent structures (particularly later in the disease process)
- Generally not painful

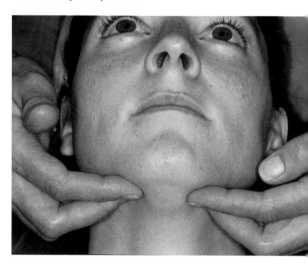

- Palpate the submandibular area - instruct the patien to tilt his/her head back slightly and carefully palpate the submandibular area.

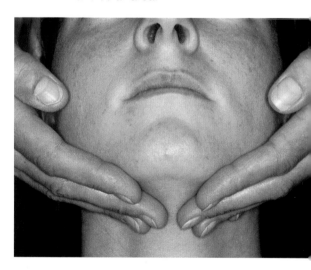

- Palpate the submental area - instruct the patient to bite together tightly and place the tongue into the palatal vault, thus tensing the mylohyoid muscle. You can then palpate the submental soft tissues against the muscle.

Examination of Intraoral Structures

Note: For oral soft tissue supported by bone (attache gingiva and mucosa of the hard palate), palpate b compressing the tissues against the bone. For tissues not supported by bone, palpate between the fingers.

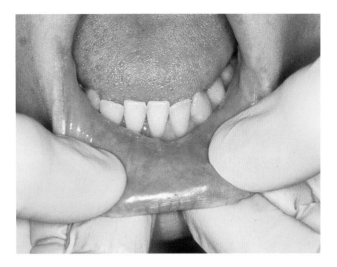

- Examine the labial and buccal mucosa - inspect the mandibular/maxillary labial mucosa and buccal mucosa. Palpate the soft tissues between the fingers.

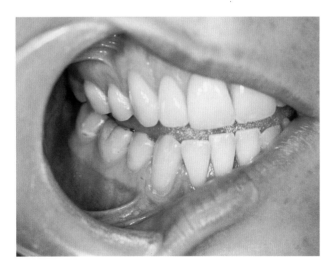

- Examine the gingiva and palatal mucosa - inspect the gingival and palatal mucosa. Palpate the tissue by compressing it against the underlying bone.

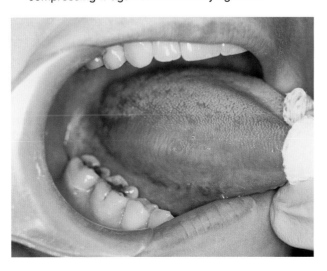

- Examine the tongue - gently hold the tip of the tongue with a piece of gauze and inspect the dorsal surface. Palpate the dorsal surface with your fingers. Move the tongue to one side and inspect the lateral border. Palpate the lateral border between the thumb and fingers. Move the tongue to the other side for inspection and palpation.

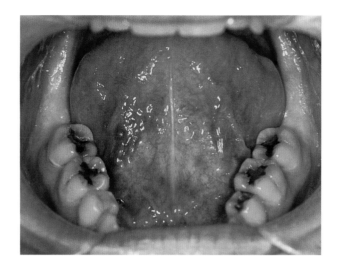

- Examine the floor of the mouth - instruct the patient to lift the tongue so that you can visualize the oral floor. Use your finger to palpate the floor of the mouth from the base of the tongue anteriorly. Palpate against the fingers of the other hand placed extraorally in the submandibular area.

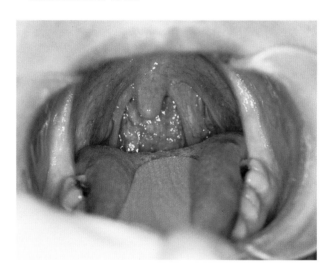

- Examine the tonsillar area and oropharynx - inspect the tonsillar area, soft palate, uvula, and oropharynx. Press down on the tongue and instruct the patient to say "ah". This causes the palatoglossal and glossopharyngeal folds to retract making it easier to visualize the area.

Carefully record all abnormal findings from the extraoral and intraoral examinations.

Note: Conventional clinical photographs or computerized digital images are both excellent methods for recording the appearance of the lesion. If you detect a lesion or lesions during the examination, you should record the following information:

INTRODUCTION *(Continued)*

- The size - measure the lesion and record the measurement

- The appearance - use the most precise descriptive terms possible when recording the appearance (a list of the most common terms is included)

- The precise location - a diagram of the oral cavity is quite useful for recording the location of a lesion (an example of a diagram of the oral cavity is included at the end of this section). Copy this diagram and have the copies available for documentation in the patient record.

- The number - is the lesion solitary or are there multiple lesions present?

For each of the images that follow, many common features will be described for each lesion illustrated. These will include:

- The color of the lesion - based on color, lesions can be classified as:

  1. Normal color - includes the range of pink characteristic of normal oral mucosal tissues taking into consideration any physiologic pigmentation that might be present

  2. White - indicates the presence of excess keratin on the epithelial surface or an accumulation of surface debris

  3. Red - indicates thinning (erosion or atrophy) of the epithelial surface or increased vascularity in the underlying submucosa

  4. Yellow - indicates presence of fatty tissue

  5. Brown, blue, or black - indicates the presence of exogenous pigment (eg, amalgam) or endogenous pigment (eg, blood products and melanin)

- Overall configuration of the lesion - flat (macular) or raised (nodular)

- Surface of the lesion - smooth (covered with intact mucosa), rough (pebbly, papillary, or corrugated), or ulcerated

- Configuration of the lesion margins - distinct or ill-defined

- Mobility of the lesion - movable or fixed (this feature helps to define how the lesion is interacting with adjacent tissue)

- Mode of attachment - broad (sessile) base or narrow (pedunculated) stalk

- Consistency - based on palpation, the lesion can be soft or firm

- Number of lesions - solitary or multiple

- Presence of bilateral symmetry - bilaterally symmetrical suggests a developmental process

- Presence of pain - a diagnostic consideration; however, because of its subjective nature, it may be of limited value

COMMONLY USED TERMS TO DESCRIBE ORAL MUCOSAL LESIONS

Bulla - a large blister (more than half a centimeter greatest dimension) on oral mucosa. Example include the oral mucosal lesions of cicatric pemphigoid and pemphigus vulgaris.

Desquamate - sloughing of the oral epithelium cause by separation from the submucosa. Desquamati lesions are often preceded by bullae. Example include the oral mucosal lesions of cicatric pemphigoid and pemphigus vulgaris.

Ecchymosis - an area of oral submucosal hemorrhag greater than 2 centimeters in greatest dimensio Oral ecchymoses are usually caused by trauma.

Endophytic - an oral mucosal lesion that extends in the adjacent tissues. Endophytic lesions are chara teristically indurated. Oral squamous cell car nomas often produce endophytic lesions.

Erosion - thinning of the epithelial surface of or mucosa. Erosions are characteristically re (erythematous) in color. Erosive lichen planus is a example.

Erythematous - an oral mucosal lesion that is red color. The red color can result from erosion of th epithelial surface of the lesions (eg, erosive liche planus), or from an increase in the number of bloc vessels in the lesion (eg, pyogenic granuloma).

Exophytic - an oral mucosal lesion that extends outwa from the surface of the adjacent mucosa. Squ mous papillomas are characteristically exophytic.

Indurated - an oral mucosal lesion that is firm to palp tion. An ulcer with indurated margins is a characte istic clinical presentation of oral squamous ce carcinoma.

Keratosis (Callous) - an adherent (cannot be wiped o white patch caused by excess keratin on the epithe lial surface of oral mucosa. Keratoses are chara teristically white in color. Frictional keratosis ar smoking-related leukoplakia are examples.

Macule - a flat, circumscribed, pigmented lesion on or mucosa. The lesion is not elevated. Example include amalgam tattoo and oral melanotic macul

Nodule - an elevated circumscribed lesion on or mucosa. Irritation fibroma is an example of nodule.

Papillary - an oral mucosal lesion with a surfac composed of numerous blunted projections. Inflam matory papillary hyperplasia is an example.

Papule - a slightly elevated circumscribed lesion on oral mucosa. Melanocytic nevus is an example of a papule.

Pedunculated - an oral mucosal lesion that is attached to the adjacent mucosa by a narrow stalk. Squamous papilloma is characteristically attached by a narrow stalk.

Petechiae - small hemorrhages in the oral submucosa. Petechiae appear clinically as small erythematous spots on the affected mucosa. Oral mucosal petechial hemorrhages are seen in infectious mononucleosis.

Pseudomembrane - a nonadherent (can be wiped off) accumulation of necrotic debris on the surface of an oral ulcer. Pseudomembranous are usually white to yellow in color. Pseudomembranous candidiasis and mucous patches of secondary syphilis are examples of oral lesions which have a pseudomembrane on their surface.

Sessile - an oral mucosal lesion that is attached to the adjacent mucosa by a broad base. Irritation fibroma is characteristically attached by a broad base.

Ulcer - a localized area of complete loss of oral epithelium. Submucosal connective tissue is exposed at the base of the ulcer. Examples include traumatic ulcers and recurrent aphthous ulcers.

Verrucous - an oral mucosal lesion with a surface composed of numerous elongated projections. The projections are commonly white in color because of hyperkeratosis. Verrucous carcinoma is an example.

Vesicle - a small blister (less than half a centimeter in greatest dimension) on oral mucosa. Examples include the initial lesions of recurrent intraoral herpes and herpangina.

ESTABLISHING A DIFFERENTIAL DIAGNOSIS

For some oral mucosal lesions, a precise diagnosis can be made based solely on patient history and clinical presentation and no additional diagnostic procedures are necessary.

However, many lesions share similar clinical features. For these lesions, it is necessary to formulate a clinical differential diagnosis. A clinical differential diagnosis is a list of diseases (usually no more than four or five) that fit the clinical presentation of the lesion. The disease you think is the most likely diagnosis should be listed first, the next most likely listed second, and so on.

In order to determine the final diagnosis, additional diagnostic procedures may be necessary. These procedures most often require removal of some or all of the lesion for microscopic examination. Diagnostic procedures include conventional biopsy, brush biopsy, and exfoliative cytology.

DIAGNOSTIC PROCEDURES

CONVENTIONAL BIOPSY

Conventional biopsy is the microscopic examination of tissue removed from an area of suspected disease. The purpose is to establish an accurate diagnosis so that the disease can be appropriately treated.

A conventional biopsy is indicated when:

- Clinical examination fails to lead to a precise diagnosis.
- A lesion fails to respond to conservative therapy within a reasonable period of time.
- A lesion is thought to be premalignant.
- A lesion exhibits clinical features of malignancy.

Incisional Biopsy

- Incisional biopsy is the surgical removal of only a sample of the lesion for the purpose of microscopic examination.
- Once a microscopic diagnosis has been made, it may be necessary to remove the remainder of the lesion.

Excisional Biopsy

- Excisional biopsy is the removal of the entire lesion with a margin of clinically uninvolved tissue.
- The procedure is meant to be both diagnostic and therapeutic.
- If microscopic examination shows that some of the lesion remains, additional surgery may be necessary.

PUNCH BIOPSY FOR ORAL MUCOSAL LESIONS

- Punch biopsy is a convenient method for performing incisional biopsies of oral mucosal lesions.
- This technique employs a disposable instrument called a biopsy punch that makes a circular incision.
- A disposable biopsy punch with a diameter of 4 mm is preferred for incisional biopsies of most oral mucosal lesions.

Instruments / Supplies Needed to Perform a Punch Biopsy

- Local anesthetic
- Surgical pack with appropriate sterile drapes and gauze
- Disposable biopsy punch (4 mm diameter punch preferred)
- Scalpel with a number 15 surgical blade, small scissors, tissue forceps, and hemostats
- Appropriate fixative (10% neutral buffered formalin for routine histopathologic examination and Michel's fluid for direct immunofluorescent studies)

INTRODUCTION *(Continued)*

Considerations for Selection of the Biopsy Site

- The biopsy site should be representative of the disease.

- Important anatomic structures in the submucosa, such as salivary gland ducts and large blood vessels, should be avoided.

- Tissue that appears to be necrotic should not be included in the biopsy specimen.

- It may be beneficial to include a margin of clinically-uninvolved tissue in the biopsy specimen.

Punch Biopsy Procedure

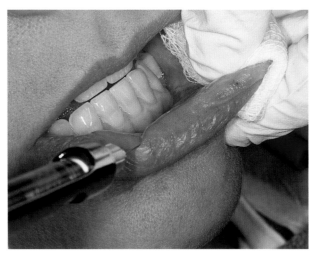

- Obtain adequate local anesthesia. Local infiltration is usually adequate. Vasoconstrictor helps to reduce hemorrhage associated with the procedure.

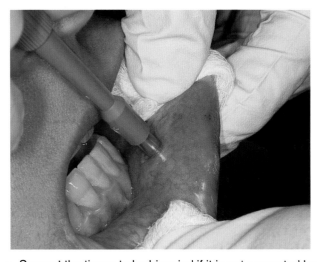

- Support the tissue to be biopsied if it is not supported by bone. If the lesion is on labial or buccal mucosa, support the tissue with your fingers. If the lesion is on the tongue, grasp the tongue with gauze to steady the biopsy site.

- Make a precise circular incision with the biopsy punch. While firmly holding the handle of the biopsy punch, place the circular blade on the lesion and rotate it while applying firm pressure. You will encounter only slight resistance from the tissue.

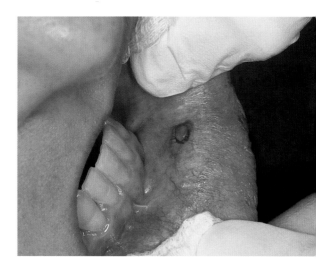

- Remove the biopsy punch to evaluate the depth of th incision. For superficial lesions, you will only need t penetrate the tissue a few millimeters. A rim of bleedin around the incision indicates that you have penetrate the epithelium. Lesions located in the submucosa w usually require a deeper incision.

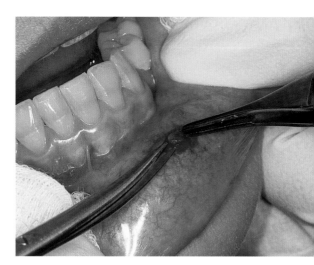

- Separate the base of the specimen from the underlyin tissue. Gently grasp the edge of the specimen wit tissue forceps and separate the base using small scis sors or a scalpel with a number 15 blade.

- Control hemorrhage. In most cases, hemorrhage can b controlled by placing sterile gauze on the biopsy sit and applying firm pressure. More persistent hemol rhage can be controlled with the application of a topica anticoagulant.

- Properly fix the tissue specimen. Place the tissue spec imen epithelium-side down on a small piece of stit paper. Allow a few seconds for the tissue to adhere t the paper and then gently place the paper in a containe with the appropriate fixative.

Postoperative Instructions for the Patient

- Maintain pressure on the biopsy site with sterile gauze until bleeding has stopped.
- Avoid injury to the biopsy site from chewing food or tooth brushing.
- Gently rinse with warm saline several times a day.
- Over-the-counter nonsteroidal anti-inflammatory medications are usually sufficient to relieve postoperative pain.

ORAL BRUSH BIOPSY

- Oral brush biopsy is the removal of all layers of the epithelium (including the basal cell layer) using a biopsy brush (a small brush with very firm bristles).
- In contrast to conventional exfoliative cytology which only provides cells from the surface of the lesion, brush biopsy generates a transepithelial specimen.
- If abnormal epithelial cells are detected, a conventional biopsy is indicated.

Indications for Oral Brush Biopsy

- Brush biopsy is especially suited for the early detection of precancerous and cancerous oral mucosal lesions.

Advantages of Oral Brush Biopsy

- Requires only a few instruments and supplies
- Easy to perform
- Well tolerated by patient
- Associated with little or no morbidity

Limitations of Oral Brush Biopsy

- Since only individual cells are examined, they cannot be evaluated in their proper tissue relationships.
- If atypical epithelial cells are detected, a conventional biopsy is indicated to confirm the diagnosis.

Instruments / Supplies for Oral Brush Biopsy

- Biopsy brush
- Coated glass microscope slides
- Commercially-available fixative

Oral Brush Biopsy Procedure

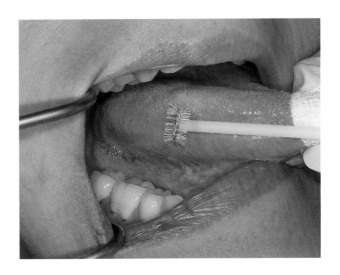

- Place the biopsy brush against the surface of the lesion and turn the brush using firm pressure 5-10 rotations.

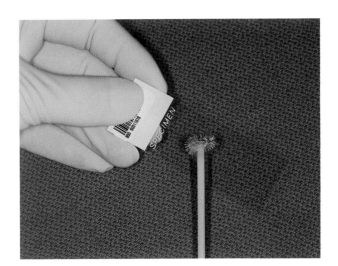

- Transfer the cellular material to a glass slide by rotating the brush on the slide. Transfer as much cellular material as possible covering the entire surface of the slide.
- Immediately coat the glass slide with fixative. Allow it to dry for 15-20 minutes.

ORAL EXFOLIATIVE CYTOLOGY

- Oral exfoliative cytology is the microscopic examination of cells from the surface of an oral mucosal lesion.
- Oral exfoliative cytology is a useful adjunct in the diagnosis of surface lesion of oral mucosa.

Indications for Oral Exfoliative Cytology

- Premalignant/malignant lesions (dysplasia, carcinoma-in-situ)

- Vesiculoulcerative diseases (herpes simplex virus, varicella zoster virus)

- Superficial fungal infections (candidiasis, geotrichosis)

Advantages of Oral Exfoliative Cytology

- Requires only a few instruments and supplies

- Easy to perform

- Well tolerated by the patient

- Associated with no morbidity

Limitations of Oral Exfoliative Cytology

- Because only surface cells are examined, the disease process must involve the mucosal surface.

- Since only individual cells are examined, the cells cannot be evaluated in their proper tissue relationships.

- If atypical epithelial cells are detected, a conventional biopsy is indicated to confirm the diagnosis.

Instruments / Supplies

- Sterile gauze

- Coated glass microscope slides

- Tongue blade, cement spatula, wax spatula (or other suitable instrument)

- Fixative (commercially-available fixative, hair spray, or isopropyl alcohol)

Procedure for Oral Exfoliative Cytology

- Select the site to obtain material for cytopathologic examination.

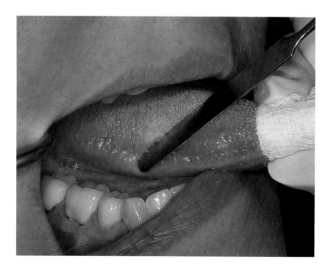

- If the lesion is on labial or buccal mucosa, suppo these structures with your fingers.

- If the lesion is on the tongue, use sterile gauze hold the tongue securely.

- Use the tongue blade, cement spatula, wax spatul or other suitable instrument to remove the cells be examined to be used on edge in a scrapir motion.

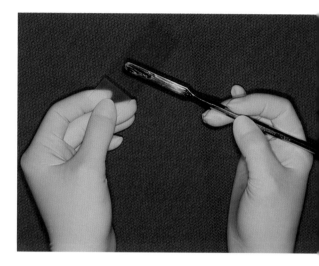

- Spread the cells on a glass slide.

- Immediately coat the slide with commerciall available fixative or hair spray, or immerse th slide in isopropyl alcohol and remove quickly.

DIRECT OPTICAL FLUORESCENCE VISUALIZATION

- Direct optical fluorescence visualization is th process of examining tissue directly with the huma eye to assess its autofluorescence properties. I order to detect the fluorescent pattern of the tissue it must be exposed to a light of specific wavelengt and intensity that excites the cells, and viewe through special filters that remove all unwanted ligl normally reflected from the tissue.

- The fluorescent pattern produced by the cells enable the clinician to differentiate between tissues con posed of normal cells and abnormal tissue, specifical premalignant and malignant epithelial neoplasm:

- In the oral cavity, direct optical fluorescence visual zation is accomplished using the VELscope, a han held, field-of-view device that provides the clinicia with an easy-to-use, adjunctive, screening instrumer for early detection of oral premalignant and malignar lesions.

The device emits a safe blue light into the oral cavity which excites cells beneath the epithelial surface causing them to fluoresce. Tissue composed of normal cells emits an apple-green fluorescence, while abnormal tissue exhibits a loss of fluorescence and appears dark.

Indications for Use of Direct Optical Fluorescence Visualization (VELscope)

- The VELscope is indicated as an adjunct to routine oral mucosal examination procedures and to aid in early clinical detection of oral premalignant and malignant lesions.

- The VELscope can also be used to evaluate the oral mucosa for possible recurrent disease of patients with a history of oral cancer.

Advantages of Direct Optical Fluorescence Visualization (VELscope)

- Simple and easy to use.
- Field-of-view technology facilitates efficient screening of oral mucosa and requires the addition of only a few minutes to the examination procedure.
- Noninvasive
- Does not require mouth rinses or tissue staining.

Limitations of Direct Optical Fluorescence Visualization (VELscope)

- If an area of concern is noted, a conventional biopsy is necessary to confirm the diagnosis of pre-malignancy or malignancy.

Instruments/Supplies Required for Direct Optical Fluorescence Visualization (VELscope)

- The VELscope Light Source Unit and Viewing Hand-piece
- Disposable asepsis barriers, cheek retractor, and 2 x 2 gauze
- Safety glasses for the patient

Visually Enhanced Vision Scope Procedure

- Conduct a thorough extraoral and intraoral exam.

  Place asepsis barriers and cheek retractor on the Viewing Handpiece.

  Instruct the patient to put on the safety glasses.

- Dim the operatory lights to optimize visualization of the oral mucosa.

- Place the Viewing Handpiece 5-10 cm (2-4 inches) from the patient's mouth.

- Illuminate the patient's oral cavity with the blue light emitted by the VELscope and repeat the intra-oral examination. The cheek retractor and 2 x 2 gauze can be used to help manipulate and retract the patient's tongue and buccal mucosa.

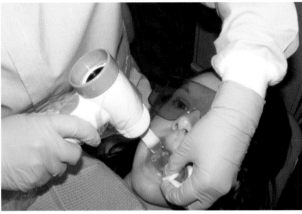

(Courtesy of Scott Benjamin)

- When viewed through the VELscope, normal tissue exhibits apple-green fluorescence, while abnormal tissue exhibits loss of fluorescence and appears dark.

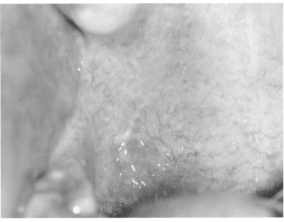

(Courtesy of the British Columbia Oral Cancer Prevention Program)

White Light Negative Lesion

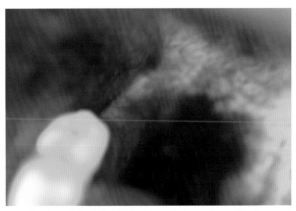

(Courtesy of the British Columbia Oral Cancer Prevention Program)

VELscope Positive Lesion

Patient Name _____ Date _____

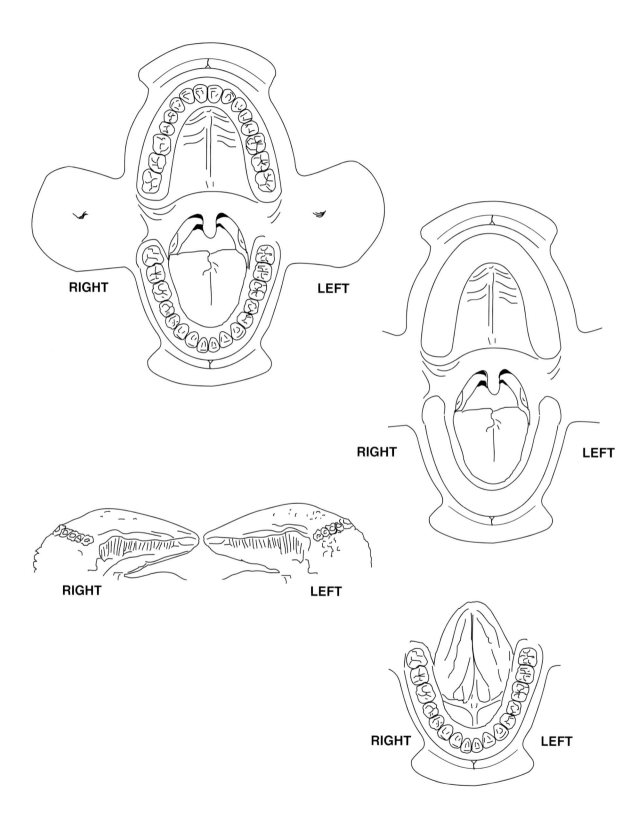

RIGHT

LEFT

RIGHT

LEFT

RIGHT

LEFT

RIGHT

LEFT

WHITE LESIONS

GENERAL PRINCIPLES

- Oral mucosal lesions can appear white because of thickening of the epithelium (acanthosis), the production of excess keratin on the epithelial surface (hyperkeratosis), or accumulations of surface organisms or debris (pseudomembranes).

- The term *leukoplakia* means a white plaque or patch that is adherent to the mucosal surface (it will not rub off).

- Because it is not possible to predict the biologic behavior of a leukoplakia based only on its clinical appearance, some other diagnostic procedure (conventional biopsy, brush biopsy, or exfoliative cytology) is often necessary to determine if the lesion is premalignant or malignant.

LIST OF DISEASES

Leukoedema 16
White Sponge Nevus 17
Fordyce's Granules 18
White Hairy Tongue 19
Frictional Keratosis 20
Acute Pseudomembranous Candidiasis 22
Chronic Hyperplastic Candidiasis 24
Cinnamon Oil Allergy 26
Reticular and Plaque-Type Lichen Planus 28
Hairy Leukoplakia 29
Smoking-Related Leukoplakia 30
Smokeless Tobacco Keratosis 31
Oral Submucous Fibrosis 32
Nicotinic Stomatitis 33
Actinic Cheilitis 34

LEUKOEDEMA

ETIOLOGY

- A developmental variation caused by thickening of the epithelium and the accumulation of edema fluid within individual epithelial cells (intracellular edema)

TYPICAL VISUAL CUES

- Adherent white opalescent thickening often with a filmy corrugated surface

- Occurs bilaterally on buccal mucosa

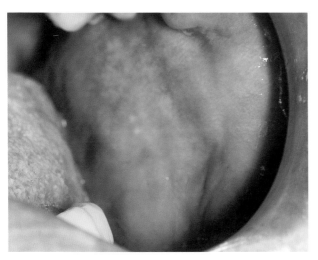

Leukoedema on the buccal mucosa (stretching the mucosa causes the white appearance to diminish)

OTHER USEFUL CLINICAL INFORMATION

- Painless
- Persistent

DIFFERENTIAL DIAGNOSIS

- Frictional keratosis
- Plaque-type lichen planus
- White sponge nevus
- Smokeless tobacco keratosis

DIAGNOSTIC STEPS

- Careful examination of the buccal mucosa

- The lesions do not rub off; however, gentle stretching of the involved mucosa causes the opalescent appearance and surface corrugations to diminish

TREATMENT RECOMMENDATIONS

- No treatment necessary

FOLLOW-UP

- Observe periodically to ensure that other mucosal changes are not present within an overlay of leukoedema

CLINICAL SIGNIFICANCE

- Leukoedema is an innocuous condition
- It is more apparent in individuals with dark skin

WHITE SPONGE NEVUS

SYNONYMS

- Familial White Folded Dysplasia

ETIOLOGY

- An autosomal-dominant genetic defect that causes thickening of the affected oral mucosa

TYPICAL VISUAL CUES

- Diffuse, thickened, corrugated, white lesions

- Occurs bilaterally on buccal mucosa

- Occasionally involves tongue, floor of the mouth, and labial mucosa

OTHER USEFUL CLINICAL INFORMATION

- Painless

- Persistent

- Usually presents during early childhood

- A parent may exhibit similar lesions

- May also involve mucosa of the larynx, esophagus, anus, and vagina

DIFFERENTIAL DIAGNOSIS

- Leukoedema

- Frictional keratosis

- Plaque-type lichen planus

- Chronic hyperplastic candidiasis

DIAGNOSTIC STEPS

- Microscopic examination of an incisional biopsy specimen will confirm the diagnosis

TREATMENT RECOMMENDATIONS

- No treatment necessary

CLINICAL SIGNIFICANCE

- White sponge nevus is innocuous

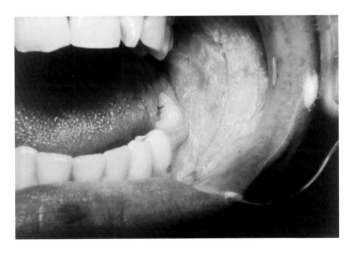

White sponge nevus on the buccal mucosa

FORDYCE'S GRANULES

SYNONYMS

- Ectopic Sebaceous Glands

ETIOLOGY

- A developmental variation caused by an accumulation of sebaceous glands in the submucosal connective tissue

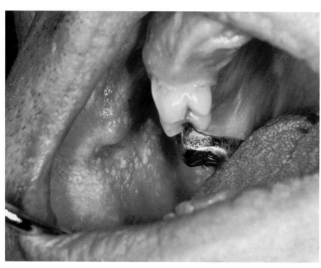

Multiple Fordyce's granules on the buccal mucosa

TYPICAL VISUAL CUES

- Multiple, small, white to yellow nodules
- Usually located on the buccal mucosa, occasionally on labial mucosa
- Commonly bilateral

OTHER USEFUL CLINICAL INFORMATION

- Painless
- Persistent

DIFFERENTIAL DIAGNOSIS

- Because of their characteristic clinical appearance Fordyce's granules are infrequently confused with other white lesions included in this section

DIAGNOSTIC STEPS

- Definitive diagnosis can usually be made on the basis of clinical presentation
- No diagnostic steps beyond recognition of clinical features

TREATMENT RECOMMENDATIONS

- No treatment necessary

CLINICAL SIGNIFICANCE

- Fordyce's granules are innocuous

WHITE HAIRY TONGUE

ETIOLOGY

- Formation of excess keratin causes elongation of the filiform papillae on the dorsal tongue

- May be infected with *Candida albicans*

TYPICAL VISUAL CUES

- Elongation of the filiform papillae

- White to yellow-tan color

- Located on the posterior dorsal tongue

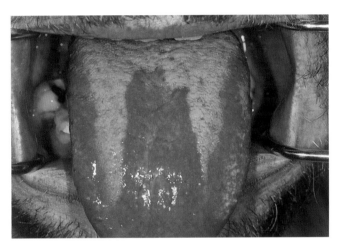

White hairy tongue

OTHER USEFUL CLINICAL INFORMATION

- Patients often have poor oral hygiene

- May complain of a bad taste

DIFFERENTIAL DIAGNOSIS

- Because of its characteristic clinical appearance, white hairy tongue is infrequently confused with other white lesions included in this section

DIAGNOSTIC STEPS

- Definitive diagnosis can usually be made on the basis of clinical presentation

- No diagnostic steps beyond recognition of clinical features

- Cytologic smear with PAS to rule out fungal involvement

TREATMENT RECOMMENDATIONS

- Elimination predisposing factors

- Cleaning the dorsal tongue with a soft toothbrush

- Treat candidiasis, if present, as in Pseudomembranous *Candida* infection

CLINICAL SIGNIFICANCE

- Despite similar names, should not be confused with the HIV-related lesion hairy leukoplakia

FRICTIONAL KERATOSIS

SYNONYMS

- Benign Hyperkeratosis

- Denture Callous or Ridge Callous (when denture-related)

ETIOLOGY

- Chronic irritation of low intensity stimulates thickening of the epithelium with the production of excess keratin (hyperkeratosis)

- The causes of chronic irritation include a broken tooth or restoration, habitual cheek- or lip-chewing, vigorous tooth brushing, hyperocclusion, or an ill-fitting denture

TYPICAL VISUAL CUES

- A circumscribed, adherent, white plaque at the site of chronic irritation

- Common sites include lateral border of tongue, buccal mucosa, attached gingiva, retromolar area, and denture-bearing mucosa

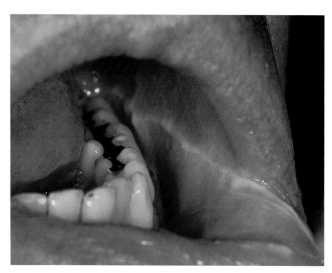

Frictional keratosis caused by habitual cheek-chewing

OTHER USEFUL CLINICAL INFORMATION

- Usually painless

- Persistent

- More common in adults

- Patient may report a history of chronic trauma

DIFFERENTIAL DIAGNOSIS

- Plaque-type lichen planus

- White sponge nevus

- Chronic hyperplastic candidiasis

- Cinnamon oil allergy

- Hairy leukoplakia (for lesions on the lateral tongue)

- Smoking-related leukoplakia

- Smokeless tobacco keratosis

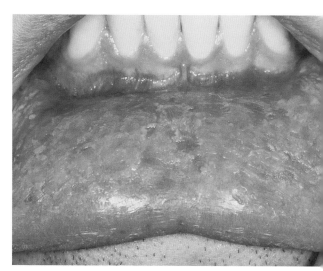

Frictional keratosis caused by habitual lip-chewing

DIAGNOSTIC STEPS

- If possible, identify and remove the presumed source of chronic mucosal irritation

- Re-evaluate the lesion in two weeks

- If it has not resolved, exfoliative cytology or brush biopsy can be performed to determine if abnormal epithelial cells are present

- A conventional biopsy may be necessary to assess the biologic potential of the lesion

20

TREATMENT RECOMMENDATIONS

- Remove all localized or generalized sources of chronic irritation (eg, repair broken tooth or restoration, or adjust an ill-fitting denture)

- Biopsy may result in removal of entire lesion

- Topical palliative treatment may hasten resolution of the lesion such as with Benzocaine (Orabase® with Benzocaine) *on page 137* or Triamcinolone (Kenalog® in Orabase® *on page 146*)

CLINICAL SIGNIFICANCE

- The lesion may represent a factitious injury associated with psychiatric illness

- Lesions in the mouths of tobacco users should be viewed with increased suspicion

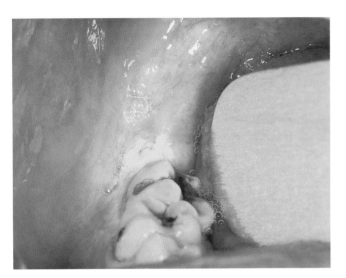

Frictional keratosis caused by hyperocclusion from a maxillary molar tooth

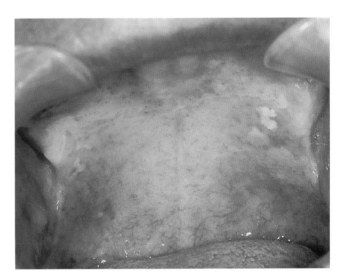

Frictional keratosis (denture callous) caused by an ill-fitting maxillary denture

ACUTE PSEUDOMEMBRANOUS CANDIDIASIS

SYNONYMS

- Thrush

ETIOLOGY

- An infection of the oral mucosa caused by the fungus, *Candida albicans* (or related species)

- The fungal organisms grow primarily on the epithelial surface

TYPICAL VISUAL CUES

- Multiple, nonadherent (will rub off), white plaques on the surface of the epithelium

- Removal of the white plaques reveals an erythematous mucosal surface

- Can occur on any oral mucosal site (most often on the buccal mucosa, tongue, and palate)

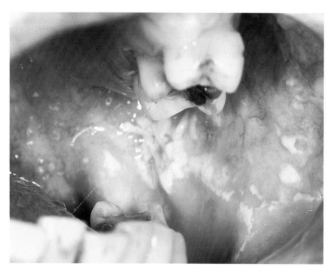

Acute pseudomembranous candidiasis on the buccal mucosa of a patient with xerostomia (the white plaques rub off)

OTHER USEFUL CLINICAL INFORMATION

- Acute onset

- Patients may complain of a dry mouth and bad taste

DIFFERENTIAL DIAGNOSIS

- Because the white plaques of acute pseudomembranous candidiasis can be rubbed off, this condition is infrequently confused with other white lesions included in this section

DIAGNOSTIC STEPS

- A cytologic smear can be prepared from the pseudomembranous debris

- Fungal organisms can be identified forming hyphae b using periodic acid-Schiff (PAS) stain

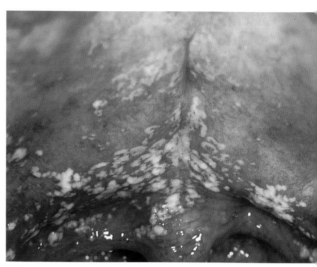

Acute pseudomembranous candidiasis on denture-bearing mucosa of the hard palate (the white plaques rub off)

TREATMENT RECOMMENDATIONS

- Antifungal agents for treatment of oral candidiasis

  - Clotrimazole (Mycelex®) oral troches *on page 13*

  - Nystatin (Mycostatin®) oral suspension *o page 144*

  - Nystatin topical *on page 144*

  - Nystatin (Mycostatin®) pastilles are no longer avail able

  - Ketoconazole cream 2% *on page 142* (not typicall advised for intraoral use)

  - Amphotericin B (Fungizone®) cream 3% *on page 136* (not typically advised for intraoral use)

- Systemic antifungal agents for chronic candidiasis

  - Ketoconazole (Nizoral®) *on page 142*

  - Fluconazole (Diflucan®) *on page 140*

  - Itraconazole (Sporanox®) capsules 100 mg *on page 142* (not usually recommended for oral infection)

FOLLOW-UP

- After a treatment course of 2-4 weeks is completed, if the lesions return when patient discontinues the anti-fungal, then underlying systemic disease such as diabetes, HIV infection, and other immunocompromised states must be reconsidered

- Persistent or recurrent episodes of acute pseudomem-branous candidiasis may indicate that the patient's immune status is compromised

CLINICAL SIGNIFICANCE

- Acute pseudomembranous candidiasis is associated with a number of predisposing factors including systemic antibiotic therapy, topical and systemic corti-costeroid therapy, dentures, chronic dry mouth, endo-crine diseases (especially diabetes mellitus), and immunosuppression

- Persistent or recurrent episodes of acute pseudomem-branous candidiasis may indicate that the patient's immune status is compromised

CHRONIC HYPERPLASTIC CANDIDIASIS

SYNONYMS

- Candidal Leukoplakia

ETIOLOGY

- Infection of the oral mucosa caused by the fungus, *Candida albicans* (or related species)

- Infected epithelium becomes hyperplastic with formation of excess surface keratin

TYPICAL VISUAL CUES

- Circumscribed, adherent (will not rub off), white plaque at the site of fungal infection

- Most often on the anterior buccal mucosa adjacent to the commissure, may occasionally involve the lateral borders of the tongue

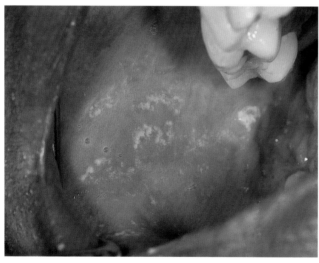

Chronic hyperplastic candidiasis on the buccal mucosa (these lesions will not rub off)

OTHER USEFUL CLINICAL INFORMATION

- Painless
- Persistent
- More common in adults

DIFFERENTIAL DIAGNOSIS

- White sponge nevus
- Frictional keratosis
- Cinnamon oil allergy
- Smoking-related leukoplakia
- Hairy leukoplakia (for lesions on the lateral tongue)
- Oral submucous fibrosis
- Plaque-type lichen planus

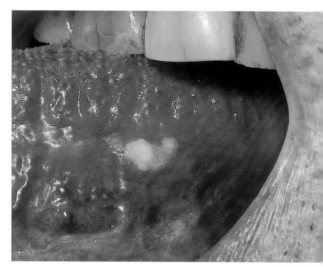

Chronic hyperplastic candidiasis on the lateral tongue (this lesion will not rub off) (biopsy revealed epithelial dysplasia)

DIAGNOSTIC STEPS

- A cytologic smear can be performed, but may not reveal the fungal organisms

- An incisional biopsy stained with periodic acid-Schiff (PAS) stain may be necessary to confirm the presence of fungal organisms

TREATMENT RECOMMENDATIONS

- Antifungal agents for treatment of oral candidiasis

   - Clotrimazole (Mycelex®) oral troches *on page 138*

   - Nystatin (Mycostatin®) oral suspension *on page 144*

   - Nystatin topical *on page 144*

- Nystatin (Mycostatin®) pastilles are no longer available

- Ketoconazole cream 2% *on page 142* (not typically advised for intraoral use)

- Amphotericin B (Fungizone®) cream 3% *on page 136* (not typically advised for intraoral use)

• Systemic antifungal agents for chronic candidiasis

  - Ketoconazole (Nizoral®) *on page 142*

  - Fluconazole (Diflucan®) *on page 140*

  - Itraconazole (Sporanox®) capsules 100 mg *on page 142* (not usually recommended for oral infection)

FOLLOW-UP

• After a treatment course of 2-4 weeks is completed, if the lesions return when patient discontinues the antifungal, then underlying systemic disease such as diabetes, HIV infection, and other immunocompromised states must be reconsidered

CLINICAL SIGNIFICANCE

• Chronic hyperplastic candidiasis may show evidence of epithelial dysplasia on microscopic examination suggesting that some of these lesions are premalignant

• Lesions in the mouths of tobacco users should be viewed with increased suspicion

CINNAMON OIL ALLERGY

SYNONYMS

- Allergic Contact Stomatitis
- Stomatitis Venenata

ETIOLOGY

- A unique mucosal allergic reaction to cinnamon oil used to flavor candy, chewing gum, toothpaste, and mouthwash.

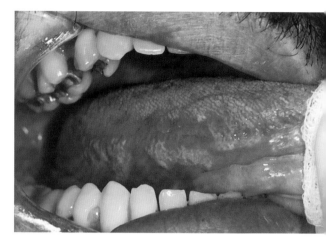

**Cinnamon oil allergy on the lateral tongue
(the patient chewed gum flavored with cinnamon oil)**

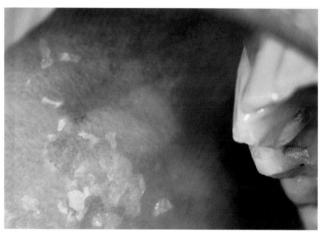

**Cinnamon oil allergy on the buccal mucosa
(the patient ate candy flavored with cinnamon oil)**

DIFFERENTIAL DIAGNOSIS

- Frictional keratosis
- Chronic hyperplastic candidiasis
- Plaque-type lichen planus
- Hairy leukoplakia
- Smoking-related leukoplakia

TYPICAL VISUAL CUES

- An adherent white plaque with a shaggy surface at the site of contact with the allergen (cinnamon oil)
- Lesions occur most often on buccal mucosa, lateral tongue, and gingiva

OTHER USEFUL CLINICAL INFORMATION

- Patient may report intermittent burning discomfort
- Patient reports onset of lesion soon after exposure to allergen

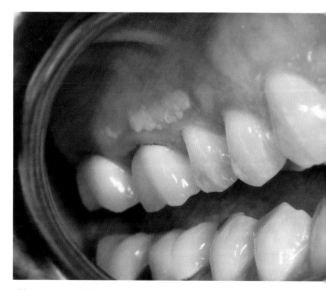

**Cinnamon oil allergy on the maxillary buccal gingiva
(the patient used a toothpaste flavored
with cinnamon oil)**

DIAGNOSTIC STEPS

- A history of cinnamon oil exposure along with the clinical presentation is often sufficient to confirm the diagnosis

- Microscopic examination if an incisional biopsy specimen will help eliminate other lesions in the differential diagnosis

TREATMENT RECOMMENDATIONS

- Lesions typically resolve within a few days after removal of the allergen

- Treatment with antihistamines such as Diphenhydramine (Benadryl® elixir *on page 140*) and topical corticosteroids such as Triamcinolone (Kenalog® in Orabase® *on page 146*)

RETICULAR AND PLAQUE-TYPE LICHEN PLANUS

ETIOLOGY

- A defect in cell-mediated immunity resulting in damage to the basal cells of oral epithelium

TYPICAL VISUAL CUES

- Reticular lichen planus appears clinically as adherent, interlacing, white striations (Wickham's striae) that occur most frequently on buccal mucosa (any other oral mucosal site can also be involved)

- Plaque-type lichen planus appears clinically as adherent, circumscribed, confluent, white plaques that occur most often on the dorsal tongue (any other oral mucosal site can also be involved)

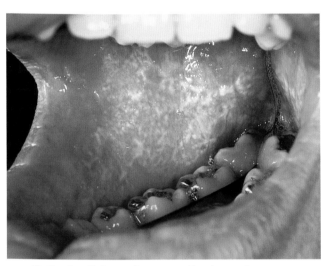

Reticular lichen planus on the buccal mucosa

OTHER USEFUL CLINICAL INFORMATION

- Usually painless
- More common in adult females

DIFFERENTIAL DIAGNOSIS

- White sponge nevus
- Frictional keratosis
- Hairy leukoplakia
- Cinnamon oil allergy
- Chronic hyperplastic candidiasis
- Leukoedema
- Smoking-related leukoplakia
- Smokeless tobacco keratosis
- Oral submucous fibrosis

DIAGNOSTIC STEPS

- If characteristic striations are present, the diagnosis can usually be made solely on the basis of clinical appearance

- In the absence of striations, microscopic examination may be necessary to confirm the diagnosis

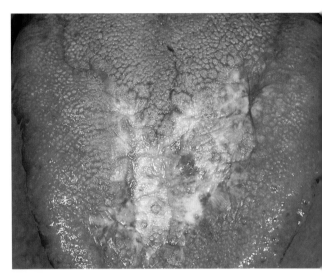

Plaque-type lichen planus on the dorsal tongue

TREATMENT RECOMMENDATIONS

- Treatment of reticular and plaque-type lichen planus is based purely on the presence of symptoms and these lesions are often/usually asymptomatic

- Patient may be being treated by a dermatologist for skin areas of lichen planus as well

- Oral lesions may require mild steroid application including Triamcinolone (Kenalog® in Orabase® on page 146) or Fluocinonide (Lidex® gel/ointment on page 141)

- Higher potency steroid applications including Dexamethasone (Decadron® on page 139) or Clobetasol (Temovate® on page 138) are not usually indicated in treatment of these mild forms of lichen planus, but can be considered if symptoms increase

CLINICAL SIGNIFICANCE

- Lesions clinically identical to lichen planus (lichenoid drug reactions) may develop from the use of a variety of medications

HAIRY LEUKOPLAKIA

ETIOLOGY

- Hyperplasia of the oral epithelium with production of excess keratin (hyperkeratosis) caused by Epstein-Barr virus infection

- The surface of the lesion is frequently infected with *Candida albicans*

- Occurs most commonly in individuals with compromised immunity secondary to human immunodeficiency virus (HIV) infection

TYPICAL VISUAL CUES

- Adherent white plaques located most often on the lateral borders of the tongue

- Surface of each lesion is characteristically corrugated or shaggy in appearance

- Typically bilateral

DIFFERENTIAL DIAGNOSIS

- Frictional keratosis

- Cinnamon oil allergy

- Plaque-type lichen planus

- Chronic hyperplastic candidiasis

- Smoking-related leukoplakia

DIAGNOSTIC STEPS

- Microscopic examination is necessary to confirm the presence of non-specific viral changes in the lesion

- Epstein-Barr virus can be identified in the lesion using a DNA probe

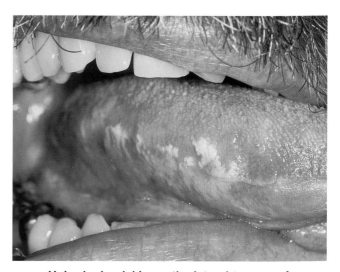

Hairy leukoplakia on the lateral tongue of an HIV-infected individual

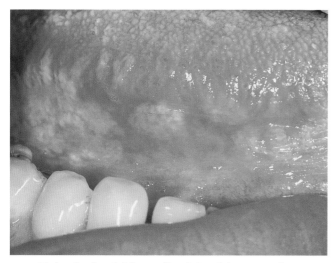

Hairy leukoplakia on the lateral tongue of an HIV-infected individual

TREATMENT RECOMMENDATIONS

- Some patients respond to high-dose Acyclovir (Zovirax® *on page 134*); lesions often recur when treatment is stopped

OTHER USEFUL CLINICAL INFORMATION

- Usually painless

- Persistent

- More common in young adult males

CLINICAL SIGNIFICANCE

- An HIV-infected individual with hairy leukoplakia is likely to develop Acquired Immunodeficiency Syndrome (AIDS) within two years

SMOKING-RELATED LEUKOPLAKIA

SYNONYMS

- Tobacco-Associated Leukoplakia
- Idiopathic Leukoplakia

ETIOLOGY

- Chronic exposure to the chemical carcinogens generated by burning tobacco

TYPICAL VISUAL CUES

- Circumscribed, adherent, white plaques that vary in size, thickness, and surface configuration
- Occur most often on lower lip, buccal mucosa, and gingiva
- Lesions on the ventral tongue and floor of the mouth are more likely to show microscopic evidence of premalignancy or malignancy

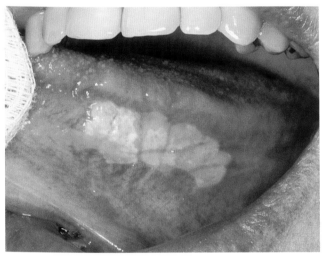

Smoking-related leukoplakia on the ventral tongue (biopsy revealed epithelial dysplasia)

OTHER USEFUL CLINICAL INFORMATION

- Painless
- Persistent
- Patient reports a history of smoking (cigarettes, cigars, and pipes)

DIFFERENTIAL DIAGNOSIS

- Frictional keratosis
- Chronic hyperplastic candidiasis
- Cinnamon oil allergy
  Plaque-type lichen planus

DIAGNOSTIC STEPS

- Routine exfoliative cytology or brush biopsy can be used to determine if abnormal epithelial cells are present
- Conventional biopsy is indicated if abnormal epithelial cells are identified or if the lesion persists

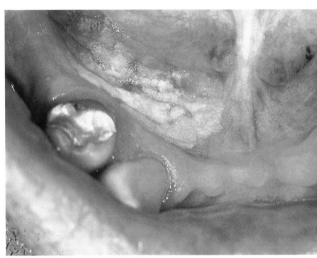

Smoking-related leukoplakia on the floor of the mouth (biopsy revealed carcinoma *in situ*)

TREATMENT RECOMMENDATIONS

- The patient should be counseled to stop smoking
- If the lesion regresses, the patient should be re-evaluated at regular intervals
- If the lesion does not regress, it should be excised and submitted for microscopic examination
- If microscopic evidence of premalignancy or malignancy is discovered, more extensive therapy is indicated
- The patient should be re-evaluated at regular intervals for other oral mucosal changes

CLINICAL SIGNIFICANCE

- Smoking-related leukoplakia in the floor of the mouth (sublingual leukoplakia) has the highest incidence of malignant transformation
- It is not possible to determine, based on clinical appearance alone, which areas of leukoplakia are premalignant or malignant
- Lesions that appear innocuous clinically may show microscopic evidence of malignant transformation

SMOKELESS TOBACCO KERATOSIS

SYNONYMS

- Tobacco Pouch Keratosis

ETIOLOGY

- Chronic exposure to chemical carcinogens liberated from smokeless tobacco (chewing tobacco and moist snuff)

TYPICAL VISUAL CUES

- Circumscribed, adherent, white plaques of varying thickness usually with a corrugated surface

- Most commonly on the mandibular labial or buccal vestibule (at the site where the smokeless tobacco is placed)

- Often associated with recession of labial gingiva adjacent to mandibular anterior teeth

OTHER USEFUL CLINICAL INFORMATION

- Painless
- Persistent
- Patient reports a history of smokeless tobacco use

DIFFERENTIAL DIAGNOSIS

- Frictional keratosis
- Chronic hyperplastic candidiasis
- Cinnamon oil allergy
- Leukoedema
- Plaque-type lichen planus
- Oral submucous fibrosis

DIAGNOSTIC STEPS

- Routine exfoliative cytology or brush biopsy can be used to determine if abnormal epithelial cells are present

- Conventional biopsy is indicated if abnormal cells are identified or if the lesion persists

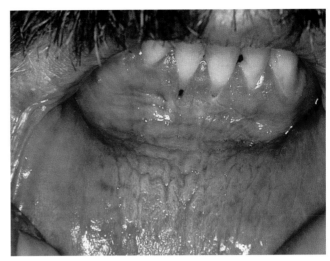

Smokeless tobacco keratosis on the mandibular labial mucosa of an individual who uses moist snuff (note the recession of the labial gingiva)

TREATMENT RECOMMENDATIONS

- The patient should be counseled to stop using smokeless tobacco

- If the lesions regress within a few weeks, periodic re-evaluation is indicated

- Lesions which show any dysplastic changes or frank microscopic evidence of malignant transformation should be referred to an oncologist for management and excised

- The patient should be re-evaluated at regular intervals for other oral mucosal changes

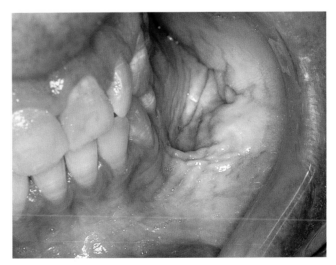

Smokeless tobacco keratosis on the buccal mucosa of an individual who uses moist snuff

CLINICAL SIGNIFICANCE

- Persistent lesions can develop into verrucous carcinoma

ORAL SUBMUCOUS FIBROSIS

ETIOLOGY

- Caused by the habitual chewing of betal quid (areca nut, slake lime, and tobacco wrapped in betal leaf)

TYPICAL VISUAL CUES

- Typically affects posterior buccal mucosa at the site of betal quid exposure

- Affected mucosa exhibits diffuse white thickening

- May occasionally involve tongue and soft palate

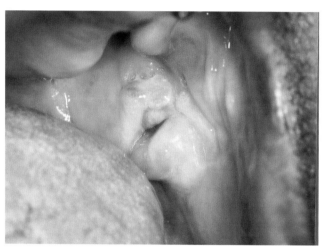

**Oral submucous fibrosis
(the patient had a 30-year history of betal quid chewing)**

OTHER USEFUL CLINICAL INFORMATION

- More common in adult males from Southeast Asia and India

- Underlying connective tissue is very firm to palpation

- Patient may have difficulty opening his mouth

- Affected mucosa may be painful

DIFFERENTIAL DIAGNOSIS

- Smoking-related leukoplakia

- Smokeless tobacco keratosis

- Plaque-type lichen planus

- Chronic hyperplastic candidiasis

DIAGNOSTIC STEPS

- Conventional biopsy is indicated to determine if the lesion is premalignant

TREATMENT RECOMMENDATIONS

- The patient should be counseled to stop using beta quid

- Persistent lesions require surgical therapy

FOLLOW-UP

- Careful periodic re-evaluation

CLINICAL SIGNIFICANCE

- Oral submucous fibrosis can develop into squamous cell carcinoma

NICOTINIC STOMATITIS

SYNONYMS

- Smoker's Palate

ETIOLOGY

- Chronic exposure to the heat liberated from burning tobacco (most often associated with pipe and cigar smoking)

TYPICAL VISUAL CUES

- Diffuse, white, thickening of the palatal mucosa with interspersed, elevated white papules each with a red central depression (the white papules with red centers are the inflamed openings of minor salivary glands)

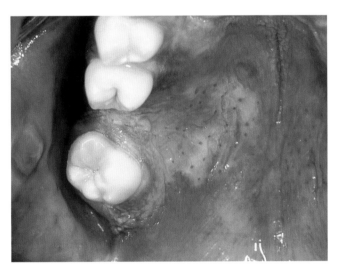

Nicotinic stomatitis on the hard palate of a cigar smoker

OTHER USEFUL CLINICAL INFORMATION

- Usually painless
- Persistent
- Patient reports a history of pipe and/or cigar smoking

DIFFERENTIAL DIAGNOSIS

- Because of its location and characteristic clinical appearance, nicotinic stomatitis is infrequently confused with other white lesions included in this section

DIAGNOSTIC STEPS

- A definitive diagnosis can usually be made on the basis of clinical presentation
- Microscopic examination may be performed to confirm the diagnosis

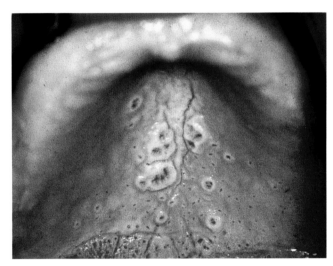

Nicotinic stomatitis on the hard palate of a pipe smoker

TREATMENT RECOMMENDATIONS

- The patient should be counseled to stop smoking
- Once the patient stops smoking, the lesions usually regress
- The patient should be re-evaluated at regular intervals for other oral mucosal changes

CLINICAL SIGNIFICANCE

- Nicotinic stomatitis has a minimal risk of malignant transformation

ACTINIC CHEILITIS

SYNONYMS

- Actinic Cheilosis

ETIOLOGY

- Chronic exposure to ultraviolet radiation from sunlight

TYPICAL VISUAL CUES

- Irregular, diffuse, adherent, white thickening of the involved epithelium

- Occurs on the vermilion of the lower lip

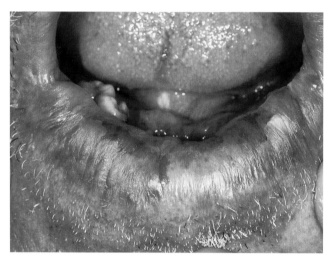

Actinic cheilitis on the lower lip of an elderly man

OTHER USEFUL CLINICAL INFORMATION

- Usually painless

- Persistent

- More common in older males

- More common in individuals with a light complexion with a history of chronic sun exposure

DIFFERENTIAL DIAGNOSIS

- Frictional keratosis

- Smoking-related leukoplakia

- Plaque-type lichen planus

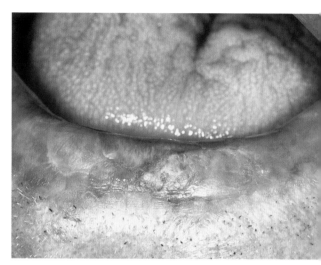

A squamous cell carcinoma arising in a pre-existing actinic cheilitis

DIAGNOSTIC STEPS

- Conventional biopsy may be necessary to confirm th diagnosis

TREATMENT RECOMMENDATIONS

- The patient should be instructed to use a sunscreen

- If the lesions persist, a biopsy should be performed t evaluate malignant potential

- If the presence of carcinoma is confirmed, more exter sive surgical therapy is indicated

CLINICAL SIGNIFICANCE

- Squamous cell carcinoma develops in approximatel 10% of cases

RED LESIONS

GENERAL PRINCIPLES

* Oral mucosal lesions can appear red because the epithelium is thinner than normal (atrophic), because there are more blood vessels in the submucosa, or because there is bleeding into the submucosal tissues.

* Atrophic oral mucosal lesions are frequently associated with burning discomfort.

* Red oral mucosal lesions associated with smoking (erythroplakias) are especially worrisome because they often exhibit microscopic evidence of premalignancy.

LIST OF DISEASES

Erythematous Candidiasis (Acute and Chronic) 36
Angular Cheilitis 38
Erythroplakia 39
Stomatitis Areata Migrans 40
Mucosal Allergy 41
Fissured Tongue 42
Atrophic Glossitis 43
Foreign Body Gingivitis 44
Plasma Cell Gingivitis 45
Median Rhomboid Glossitis 46
Lingual Varicosities 47
Submucosal Hemorrhages 48

ERYTHEMATOUS CANDIDIASIS (Acute and Chronic)

SYNONYMS

- Atrophic Candidiasis (Acute and Chronic)

- Antibiotic Stomatitis/Sore Mouth (Acute Erythematous Candidiasis)

- Denture Stomatitis/Sore Mouth (Chronic Erythematous Candidiasis)

OTHER USEFUL CLINICAL INFORMATION

- Acute erythematous stomatitis is commonly associated with localized burning discomfort (can cause burning mouth syndrome)

ETIOLOGY

- An infection of the oral mucosa caused by the fungus, *Candida albicans* (or related species)

- Systemic broad spectrum antibiotics predispose to acute erythematous candidiasis (antibiotic stomatitis/ sore mouth)

- Ill-fitting dentures predispose to chronic erythematous candidiasis (denture stomatitis/sore mouth)

- Other predisposing factors include immunosuppression (including cancer chemotherapy), radiation therapy, and chronic dry mouth

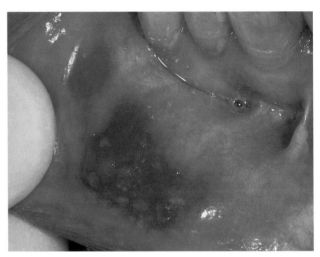

Acute erythematous candidiasis on the mandibular labial mucosa of an individual who is taking a broad spectrum antibiotic

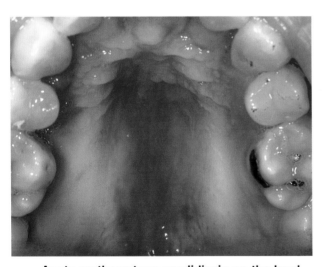

Acute erythematous candidiasis on the hard palate of an individual who is taking a broad spectrum antibiotic

DIFFERENTIAL DIAGNOSIS

- Atrophic glossitis

- Erythroplakia

- Stomatitis areata migrans

- Mucosal allergy

TYPICAL VISUAL CUES

- Generalized mucosal erythema

- Acute erythematous candidiasis frequently affects the dorsal tongue and palate

- Chronic erythematous candidiasis commonly affects denture-bearing mucosa (especially the hard palate)

DIAGNOSTIC STEPS

- A cytologic smear can be prepared from material on the lesion surface and stained with periodic acid-Schiff stain to identify the fungal organisms

TREATMENT RECOMMENDATIONS

- For denture stomatitis/sore mouth, reline existing denture or fabricate a new denture

- Appropriate antifungal therapy

- Antifungal agents for treatment of oral candidiasis

  - Clotrimazole (Mycelex®) oral troches *on page 138*
  - Nystatin (Mycostatin®) oral suspension *on page 144*
  - Nystatin (Mycostatin®) ointment *on page 144*
  - Nystatin (Mycostatin®) pastilles are no longer available
  - Ketoconazole cream 2% (not typically advised for intraoral use) *on page 142*
  - Amphotericin B (Fungizone®) ointment (3%) (not typically advised for intraoral use) *on page 136*

- Systemic antifungal agents for chronic candidiasis

  - Ketoconazole (Nizoral®) 200 mg *on page 142*
  - Fluconazole (Diflucan®) 100 mg tablets *on page 140*
  - Itraconazole (Sporanox®) capsules 100 mg *on page 142* (not usually recommended for oral infections)

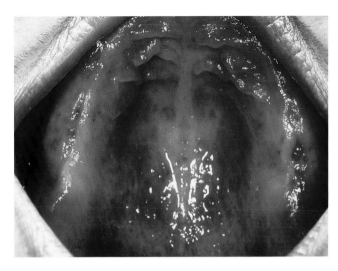

Chronic erythematous candidiasis on the denture-bearing mucosa of the maxilla (the patient had worn an ill-fitting maxillary denture for many years)

FOLLOW-UP

- After a treatment course of 2-4 weeks is completed, if the lesions return when patient discontinues the anti-fungal, then underlying systemic disease such as diabetes, HIV infection, and other immunocompromised states must be reconsidered

CLINICAL SIGNIFICANCE

- Denture stomatitis/sore mouth on the hard palate is often accompanied by inflammatory papillary hyperplasia

- Chronic infection may be associated with immunosuppression

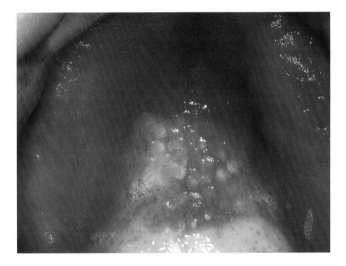

Chronic erythematous candidiasis on the denture-bearing mucosa of the maxilla

(From Newland JR, Lynch DP, and Fasser CE, *Physician Assistant*, 1983, 7(12):37-42)

ANGULAR CHEILITIS

SYNONYMS

- Perleche

ETIOLOGY

- An infection of the mucosa at the corners of the mouth caused by the fungus, *Candida albicans* (or related species)

- Other contributing factors include loss of vertical dimension (usually associated with ill-fitting dentures), bacterial infection (usually *Staphylococcus aureus*), nutritional deficiency (iron and B complex vitamins), and chronic irritation from habitual licking of the corners of the mouth

TYPICAL VISUAL CUES

- Exaggerated creases at the corners of the mouth with erythematous fissuring

- The patient may be edentulous and wear ill-fitting dentures

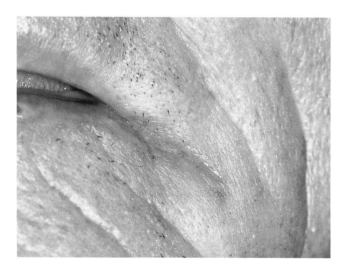

Angular cheilitis in a patient who has lost vertical dimension because of ill-fitting dentures

OTHER USEFUL CLINICAL INFORMATION

- Patients may describe burning discomfort localized to the corners of the mouth

- More common in adults

DIFFERENTIAL DIAGNOSIS

- Because of its characteristic clinical appearance angular cheilitis is infrequently confused with other erythematous lesions included in this section

DIAGNOSTIC STEPS

- A cytologic smear can be prepared from lesional material and stained with periodic acid-Schiff (PAS) stain to identify the fungal organisms

- A culture should be performed to determine if a staphylococcal infection is present

TREATMENT RECOMMENDATIONS

- Appropriate antifungal/anti-inflammatory therapy, see Nystatin/Triamcinolone Acetate *on page 145* or Iodoquinol and Hydrocortisone *on page 142*

- If the patient has lost vertical dimension because of ill-fitting dentures, new dentures should be fabricated

- Treat bacterial infection, if present

- Treat nutritional deficiency, if present

ERYTHROPLAKIA

SYNONYMS

- Erythroleukoplakia
- Speckled Leukoplakia
- Erythroplasia

ETIOLOGY

- Chronic exposure to carcinogenic components of tobacco smoke is a significant risk factor for erythroplakia
- Other factors such as chronic alcohol exposure may contribute to the development of erythroplakia

TYPICAL VISUAL CUES

- Circumscribed or ill-defined, erythematous plaques that vary in size, thickness, and surface configuration (often described as velvety in appearance)
- Occur most frequently on the floor of mouth, ventral tongue, and soft palate

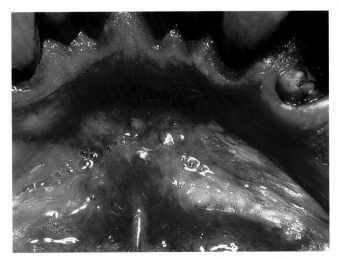

Erythroplakia on the floor of the mouth (biopsy revealed epithelial dysplasia)

OTHER USEFUL CLINICAL INFORMATION

- Painless
- Persistent
- More common in adult males
- Patient reports tobacco exposure

DIFFERENTIAL DIAGNOSIS

- Erythematous candidiasis
- Mucosal allergy

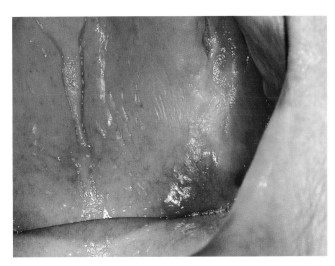

Erythroplakia on the soft palate (biopsy revealed carcinoma *in situ*)

DIAGNOSTIC STEPS

- Routine exfoliative cytology or brush biopsy can be used to determine if abnormal epithelial cells are present
- Conventional biopsy is indicated if abnormal epithelial cells are identified or if the lesion persists

TREATMENT RECOMMENDATIONS

- The patient should be counseled to stop smoking
- If microscopic evidence of premalignancy or malignancy is discovered, more extensive therapy is indicated
- The patient should be re-evaluated at regular intervals for other oral mucosal changes

CLINICAL SIGNIFICANCE

- Erythroplakia occurs less frequently than leukoplakia, but it is much more likely to exhibit microscopic evidence of dysplasia, premalignancy, or malignancy
- Many erythroplakias represent carcinoma *in situ*
- Multifocal lesions are common

STOMATITIS AREATA MIGRANS

SYNONYMS

- Erythema Migrans
- Benign Migratory Glossitis
- Geographic Tongue

ETIOLOGY

- The precise etiology of stomatitis areata migrans is unknown
- Hypersensitivity, hormonal imbalance, and emotional stress may predispose to stomatitis areata migrans in some patients

TYPICAL VISUAL CUES

- Circumscribed erythematous patches
- May be encircled with elevated hyperkeratotic (white) margins
- Occur most commonly on the dorsal and ventral tongue (other oral mucosal sites can occasionally be involved)
- May be associated with fissured tongue

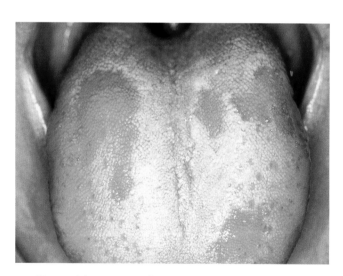

Stomatitis areata migrans on the dorsal tongue

OTHER USEFUL CLINICAL INFORMATION

- Occasionally associated with a burning sensation
- Lesions tend to move from one location to another

DIFFERENTIAL DIAGNOSIS

- Erythematous candidiasis
- Erythroplakia

DIAGNOSTIC STEPS

- A definitive diagnosis can usually be made on the basis of clinical presentation
- When clinical presentation is equivocal, microscopic examination of an incisional biopsy specimen will usually confirm the diagnosis

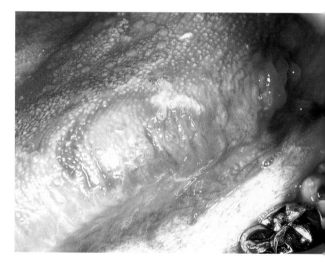

Stomatitis areata migrans on the ventral tongue

TREATMENT RECOMMENDATIONS

- Most cases are asymptomatic and require no treatment
- Symptomatic lesions can be treated with topical anti-inflammatory agents such as Triamcinolone (Kenalog® in Orabase® *on page 146*) or Fluocinonide (Lidex® *on page 141*)
- If fungal involvement is confirmed, antifungal therapy as in erythematous candidiasis, is indicated

CLINICAL SIGNIFICANCE

- There may be an increased incidence of stomatitis areata migrans in the mouths of patients with diabetes mellitus

MUCOSAL ALLERGY

SYNONYMS

- Allergic Contact Stomatitis
- Stomatitis Venenata

ETIOLOGY

- A variety of etiologic factors have been implicated in the development of mucosal allergic reactions including foods, flavoring agents, toothpastes, mouthwashes, and dental materials

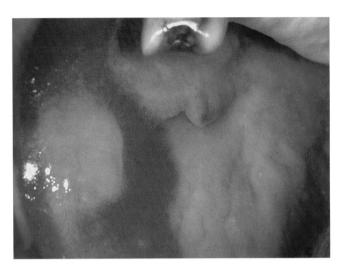

Mucosal allergy secondary to mouthwash

TYPICAL VISUAL CUES

- Circumscribed erythematous patches at the site of contact with the allergen
- Any oral mucosal site can be involved

OTHER USEFUL CLINICAL INFORMATION

- Patient may complain of localized discomfort
- Patient may report contact with offending allergen

DIFFERENTIAL DIAGNOSIS

- Atrophic glossitis
- Erythematous candidiasis
- Erythroplakia
- Stomatitis areata migrans

DIAGNOSTIC STEPS

- A definitive diagnosis can usually be made on the basis of clinical presentation and identification of the suspected allergen

TREATMENT RECOMMENDATIONS

- Removal of the suspected allergen
- Treatment with antihistamines and topical corticosteroids such as Triamcinolone (Kenalog® in Orabase® *on page 146*)

FISSURED TONGUE

SYNONYMS

- Scrotal Tongue
- Plicated Tongue

ETIOLOGY

- Precise etiology unknown
- May be the result of a genetic defect (polygenic or autosomal dominant)
- Environmental factors such as chronic dry mouth may contribute to condition

TYPICAL VISUAL CUES

- Deep fissures and grooves on the dorsal tongue
- Blunted filiform papillae
- Erythematous mucosa

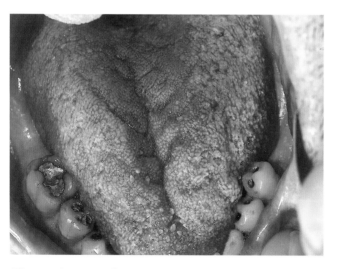

Fissured tongue in a patient with chronic xerostomia

OTHER USEFUL CLINICAL INFORMATION

- More common in adult males
- Typically asymptomatic; however, may be associated with burning discomfort
- Often associated with stomatitis areata migrans (geographic tongue)

DIFFERENTIAL DIAGNOSIS

- Because of its characteristic clinical appearance fissured tongue is infrequently confused with other white lesions included in this section

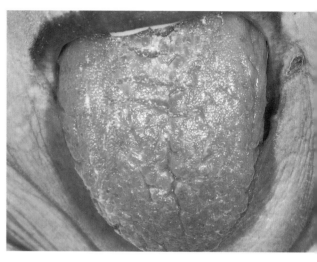

Fissured tongue in a patient with chronic xerostomia

DIAGNOSTIC STEPS

- Definitive diagnosis can usually be made on the basis of clinical presentation
- No diagnostic steps beyond recognition of clinical features

TREATMENT RECOMMENDATIONS

- Tongue brushing to keep the fissures and grooves free of debris

CLINICAL SIGNIFICANCE

- Common in patients with Down's syndrome
- A component of Melkerson-Rosenthal syndrome (fissured tongue, cheilitis granulomatosa, and unilateral facial nerve paralysis)
- Associated with chronic xerostomia

ATROPHIC GLOSSITIS

SYNONYMS

- Bald Tongue
- Beefy-Red Tongue

ETIOLOGY

- Atrophic glossitis is commonly associated with a dietary deficiency or poor absorption of nutritional components such as iron (iron deficiency anemia) and vitamin B_{12} (pernicious anemia)
- Vitamin B_{12} and iron are essential for the normal maturation of oral epithelium
- In the absence of B_{12} or iron, papillae on the dorsal surface of the tongue fail to mature properly resulting in atrophic glossitis
- Chronic dry mouth can contribute to atrophic glossitis

TYPICAL VISUAL CUES

- Focal or generalized loss of papillae on the dorsal tongue with mucosal redness
- May be accompanied by chronic dry mouth

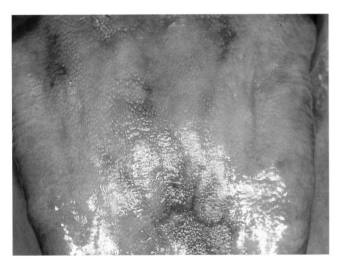

Atrophic glossitis in a patient with pernicious anemia (the patient complained of a burning tongue)

(Copyright © *Texas Dental Journal*. Used with permission)

OTHER USEFUL CLINICAL INFORMATION

- Patients with atrophic glossitis complain of a burning sensation (can cause burning mouth syndrome)
- Patients with pernicious anemia can also exhibit neurologic symptoms (especially difficulty walking)

DIFFERENTIAL DIAGNOSIS

- Erythematous candidiasis
- Stomatitis areata migrans
- Mucosal allergy
- Median rhomboid glossitis

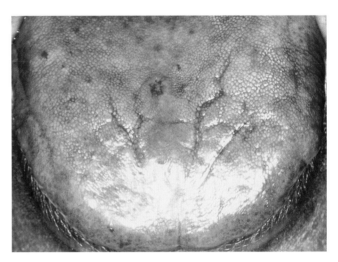

Atrophic glossitis in a patient with chronic iron deficiency anemia (the patient complained of a burning tongue)

DIAGNOSTIC STEPS

- Other indicators of chronic dry mouth should be evaluated (generalized mucosal dryness, decreased flow of parotid saliva, decreased pooled saliva in the floor of the mouth, the presence of thick saliva, increased cervical caries, and fissured tongue)
- The patient should be referred to the appropriate physician for hematologic and other studies to determine if a nutritional anemia is present

TREATMENT RECOMMENDATIONS

- Appropriate therapy for dietary deficiency or poor absorption of iron or B_{12}
- Palliation for glossitis until normal mucosa is restored

CLINICAL SIGNIFICANCE

- Iron-deficiency anemia can be associated with chronic gastric bleeding caused by gastrointestinal cancer
- Iron-deficiency anemia is a component of Plummer-Vinson syndrome
- There is an increased risk of oral and esophageal cancer in patients with Plummer-Vinson syndrome

FOREIGN BODY GINGIVITIS

SYNONYMS

- Prophy Paste Gingivitis

ETIOLOGY

- Damage to the sulcular epithelium during dental prophylaxis allows prophy paste to be embedded in the underlying connective tissue

- The prophy paste causes a foreign body inflammatory reaction

TYPICAL VISUAL CUES

- Usually involves marginal gingiva

- Solitary or multifocal distribution

- Affected gingiva red and swollen

DIFFERENTIAL DIAGNOSIS

- Plasma cell gingivitis

- Wegener's granulomatosis (for gingival lesions)

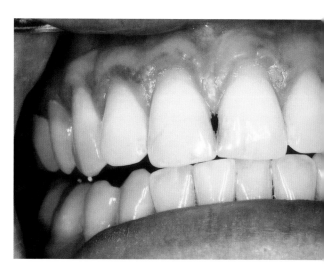

Foreign body gingivitis caused by prophy paste

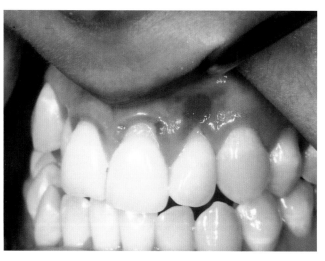

Foreign body gingivitis caused by prophy paste

DIAGNOSTIC STEPS

- Microscopic examination of an incisional biopsy spe imen may be necessary to confirm the diagnosis

TREATMENT RECOMMENDATIONS

- Topical corticosteroid therapy including Fluocinoni on page 141, in severe cases, Clobetasol page 138

- Gingivoplasty for refractory cases

OTHER USEFUL CLINICAL INFORMATION

- Usually develops soon after dental prophylaxis

- More common in adults

- May be associated with intermittent burning discomfort

CLINICAL SIGNIFICANCE

- Lesions which are similar, both clinically and micr scopically, can occasionally be seen in system diseases such as Crohn's disease, sarcoidosis, a Wegener's granulomatosis

PLASMA CELL GINGIVITIS

SYNONYMS

- Allergic Gingivostomatitis

ETIOLOGY

- An allergic (hypersensitivity) reaction to chewing gum, toothpaste, or peppers

TYPICAL VISUAL CUES

- Generalized enlargement of the maxillary and mandibular attached gingiva

- The enlarged gingiva is bright red in color

- Angular cheilitis

- Fissured tongue

DIFFERENTIAL DIAGNOSIS

- Foreign body gingivitis

- Atrophic glossitis

- Angular cheilitis

- Stomatitis areata migrans

- Mucosal allergy

DIAGNOSTIC STEPS

- A definitive diagnosis can usually be made on the basis of clinical presentation

- A biopsy may be necessary to confirm the diagnosis

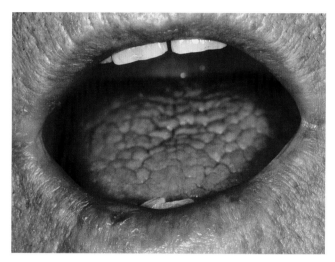

Angular cheilitis and fissured tongue in a patient with plasma cell gingivitis

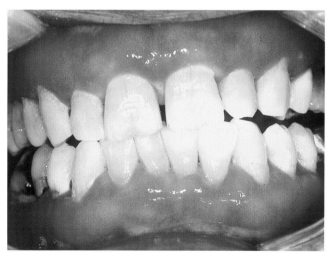

Plasma cell gingivitis secondary to toothpaste

OTHER USEFUL CLINICAL INFORMATION

- Patients with plasma cell gingivitis commonly complain of burning lips and tongue

- Patient may report contact with offending allergen

TREATMENT RECOMMENDATIONS

- Removal of all suspected allergens

- Treatment with topical corticosteroids, such as Triamcinolone (Kenalog® in Orabase® *on page 146*) is usually not necessary, but may aid in healing

- Counsel to stop chewing gum, if appropriate

MEDIAN RHOMBOID GLOSSITIS

SYNONYMS

- Median Papillary Atrophy

ETIOLOGY

- Originally thought to represent a developmental defect of the dorsal tongue

- Now considered to be a clinical manifestation of chronic erythematous candidiasis

TYPICAL VISUAL CUES

- An erythematous rhomboid-shaped area of papillary atrophy on the midline dorsal tongue

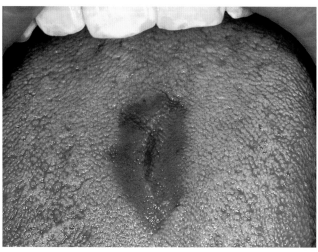

Median rhomboid glossitis on the dorsal tongue

OTHER USEFUL CLINICAL INFORMATION

- The lesions are occasionally associated with intermittent burning discomfort

- Persistent

DIFFERENTIAL DIAGNOSIS

- Atrophic glossitis

- Erythematous candidiasis

- Stomatitis areata migrans

- Mucosal allergy

DIAGNOSTIC STEPS

- Because of its characteristic clinical appearance median rhomboid glossitis is infrequently confused with other lesions

- Microscopic examination may be necessary to confirm the diagnosis

- Staining of the biopsy tissue with periodic acid-Schiff (PAS) stain will confirm the presence of fungal organisms

TREATMENT RECOMMENDATIONS

- No treatment necessary unless fungal colonization is confirmed; in that case, treat like erythematous candidiasis

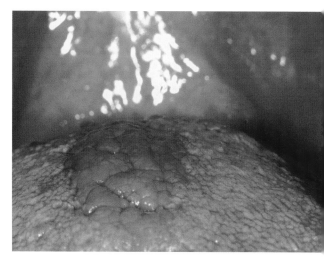

Median rhomboid glossitis on the dorsal tongue

CLINICAL SIGNIFICANCE

- Median rhomboid glossitis is occasionally confused with squamous cell carcinoma; however, this malignancy rarely occurs on the dorsal tongue

LINGUAL VARICOSITIES

SYNONYMS

- Varicose veins

ETIOLOGY

- Dilated veins caused by loss of the elasticity of the vein wall

- Commonly associated with the aging process

TYPICAL VISUAL CUES

- Commonly presents as multiple, superficial, red-purple nodules on the ventral and lateral tongue

- Occasionally presents as a solitary nodule on the ventral tongue, labial mucosa, or buccal mucosa

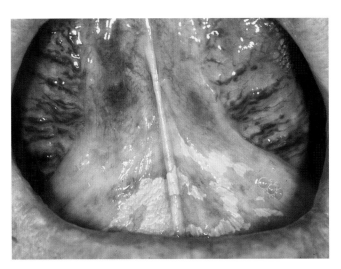

**Multiple lingual varicosities
(this patient also had a smoking-related leukoplakia
on the floor of the mouth)**

OTHER USEFUL CLINICAL INFORMATION

- Asymptomatic
- More common in elderly adults
- Multiple varicosities are compressible on palpation
- Solitary varicosity may contain a thrombus and be firm to palpation

DIFFERENTIAL DIAGNOSIS

- Because of their characteristic clinical appearance, multiple varicosities are infrequently confused with other red lesions included in this section

- A solitary varicosity may be confused with other vascular lesions such as hemangioma

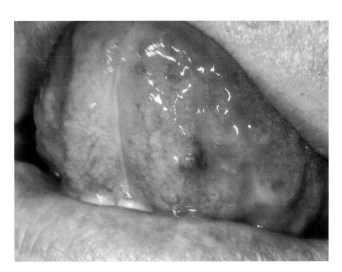

**A solitary lingual varicosity
(microscopic examination revealed the presence of a
thrombus)**

DIAGNOSTIC STEPS

- Definitive diagnosis can usually be made on the basis of clinical presentation

- No diagnostic steps beyond recognition of clinical features

TREATMENT RECOMMENDATIONS

- No treatment necessary for multiple lingual varicosities

- A varicosity which contains a thrombus may require surgical excision

CLINICAL SIGNIFICANCE

- Not associated with systemic hypertension or other cardiopulmonary diseases

SUBMUCOSAL HEMORRHAGES

SYNONYMS

- Petechiae
- Ecchymosis
- Hematoma

ETIOLOGY

- Petechiae and ecchymosis are commonly caused by suction (negative pressure) from dentures, sore throat (often associated with infectious mononucleosis), and sexual activity (fellatio)

- Hematomas are caused by more severe trauma to oral mucosa (most commonly biting injury, but occasionally iatrogenic injury)

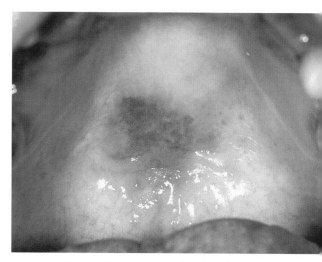

An ecchymosis on the hard palate secondary to trauma

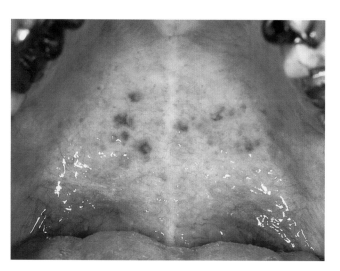

Petechial hemorrhages on the hard palate of a patient with infectious mononucleosis

DIFFERENTIAL DIAGNOSIS

- Because of their characteristic clinical appearance, petechiae are infrequently confused with other red lesions included in this section

- Ecchymoses may be confused with other diffuse red macules such as chronic erythematous candidiasis and mucosal allergy

- Hematomas may be confused with hemangiomas

TYPICAL VISUAL CUES

- Petechiae appear as multiple, small, red spots
- Ecchymoses appear as larger, more diffuse, red macules with irregular margins
- Both petechiae and ecchymoses occur most often on the palate
- Hematomas present as circumscribed, compressible, red nodules
- Hematomas occur most often on labial and buccal mucosa

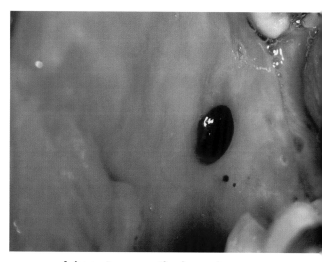

A hematoma on the buccal mucosa caused by biting injury

OTHER USEFUL CLINICAL INFORMATION

- Patient may report a positive history of mucosal injury

DIAGNOSTIC STEPS

- Definite diagnosis can usually be made on the basis of clinical presentation

- No diagnostic steps beyond recognition of clinical features

TREATMENT RECOMMENDATIONS

- Counseling with the patient about the presumed cause

- Periodic re-evaluation until the lesion(s) resolve

CLINICAL SIGNIFICANCE

- More extensive area of hemorrhage, especially those involving gingiva, can be associated with thrombocytopenia, leukemic, or bleeding disorders such as hemophilia

ULCERATED LESIONS

GENERAL PRINCIPLES

- Oral mucosal ulcers can be classified based on their extension into underlying tissues as superficial (example - aphthous ulcer) or deep-seated (example - squamous cell carcinoma).

- Many oral mucosal viral infections present initially as small blisters (vesicles), but the blisters quickly rupture to form small superficial ulcers (example - recurrent intraoral herpes).

- Individuals who wear dentures are accustomed to denture-related traumatic ulcers. As a consequence, they may ignore a malignant lesion adjacent to a denture, assuming it is denture-related and thus harmless.

- In general, if an oral mucosal ulcer persists for more than two weeks following appropriate treatment, a biopsy is indicated.

- For deep-seated lesions, the size of the ulcer may not reflect the true extent of the underlying disease (example - squamous cell carcinoma).

- Some oral mucosal ulcers are caused by infections that are contagious and thus pose an occupational risk for members of the dental team.

- All the blistering/sloughing lesions discussed in the preceding section can also present as oral mucosal ulcers.

- Oral mucosal ulcers can be associated with a variety of systemic diseases, and in some cases, they can be the initial clinical manifestation.

LIST OF DISEASES

Traumatic Ulcer 52
Aphthous Ulcers 54
Primary Herpetic Gingivostomatitis 56
Recurrent Herpes 58
Herpangina 60
Herpes Zoster 61
Primary Syphilis 62
Secondary Syphilis 63
Tuberculosis 64
Deep Fungal Infection / Histoplasmosis 65
Wegener's Granulomatosis 66
Necrotizing Ulcerative Gingivitis 67
Necrotizing Sialometaplasia 68
Ulcers Associated With Systemic Disease 69
Squamous Cell Carcinoma 70
Salivary Gland Carcinoma 71

TRAUMATIC ULCER

ETIOLOGY

- Mechanical injury to oral mucosa caused by biting, sharp foods, tooth brushing, ill-fitting dentures (denture ulcer), and iatrogenic injury during the course of dental treatment

- A self-inflicted wound associated with a psychiatric disorder is called a factitious injury

TYPICAL VISUAL CUES

- Typically, a superficial ulcer surrounded with a margin of erythematous mucosa

- The surface usually covered with a yellow pseudomembrane

- Larger traumatic ulcers called traumatic ulcerated granulomas present as deep-seated ulcers often more than 2 cm in diameter with elevated margins

- Commonly occur on the tongue, lips, and buccal mucosa (biting injury), hard palate (injury from sharp foods), and gingiva and vestibular mucosa (denture-related injury)

- Traumatic ulcerated granulomas occur most often on the lateral tongue

OTHER USEFUL CLINICAL INFORMATION

- Usually painful

- Patient may report a history of traumatic injury

- Superficial traumatic ulcers usually heal within two weeks

- Traumatic ulcerated granulomas may persist for a month or longer

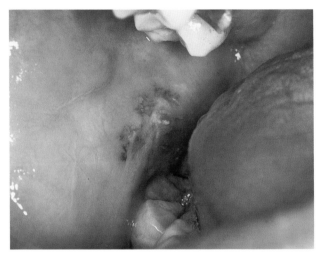

Traumatic ulcers on the buccal mucosa caused by biting injury

(From Newland JR, "Oral Ulcers," *Difficult Diagnosis 2*, Taylor RB (ed), Philadelphia, PA: WB Saunders, 1992)

DIFFERENTIAL DIAGNOSIS

- Aphthous ulcers

- Recurrent intraoral herpes

- Herpes zoster

- Hepangina

- Ulcers associated with systemic disease

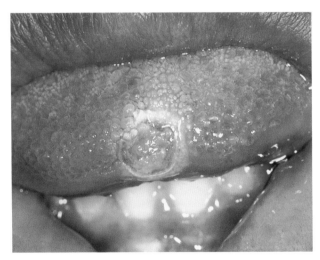

Traumatic ulcer on the tip of the tongue caused by biting injury

(From Newland JR, *Consultant*, 1989, 29:157-73.)

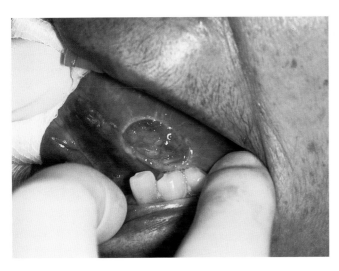

Traumatic ulcerated granuloma on the lateral tongue caused by a fractured tooth (the ulcer has been present for more than 2 months)

DIAGNOSTIC STEPS

- Determine if there is a history of trauma

- Remove suspected etiology

- Treat with palliation

- If lesion has not resolved, microscopic examination necessary to confirm diagnosis

TREATMENT RECOMMENDATIONS

- Remove etiology

- Palliation; generally lesions are self-limiting and coating with Triamcinolone (Kenalog® in Orabase® *on page 146*) may be the only requirement

CLINICAL SIGNIFICANCE

- Lesion may represent a factitious injury associated with psychiatric illness

APHTHOUS ULCERS

SYNONYMS

- Recurrent Aphthous Stomatitis
- Canker Sores

ETIOLOGY

- An immunologic defect in which both humoral and cellular immune mechanisms damage affected oral mucosa
- Physical and emotional stress appears to be a precipitating factor in many patients

TYPICAL VISUAL CUES

- Superficial ulcer with an erythematous border and a white to yellow pseudomembrane
- Classified based on their size into minor ulcers (less than 0.5 cm in diameter), major ulcers (larger than 0.5 cm in diameter), and herpetiform ulcers (clusters of small ulcers resembling the pattern of recurrent intraoral herpes)
- Typically occur on nonkeratinized mucosa (labial mucosa, buccal mucosa, ventral tongue, soft palate, tonsillar fauces, and floor of the mouth)
- Rarely occur on keratinized mucosa (attached gingiva and hard palate)
- Multiple ulcerations are common

OTHER USEFUL CLINICAL INFORMATION

- Occur with greatest frequency in young adults
- Associated with severe local discomfort
- Multiple recurrences are common

DIFFERENTIAL DIAGNOSIS

- Primary herpetic gingivostomatitis
- Recurrent intraoral herpes
- Herpes zoster
- Herpangina
- Erythema multiforme
- Traumatic ulcers
- Ulcers associated with systemic disease

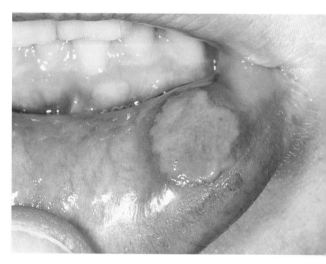

Major aphthous ulcer on the mandibular labial mucosa

(From Newland JR, "Oral Ulcers," *Difficult Diagnosis 2*, Taylor RB (ed), Philadelphia, PA: WB Saunders, 1992)

DIAGNOSTIC STEPS

- A definitive diagnosis can usually be made on the basis of clinical presentation
- A cytologic smear can be prepared from the ulcer surface and stained with Papanicolaou stain to rule out a viral etiology (there will be no evidence of viral cytopathic effect)

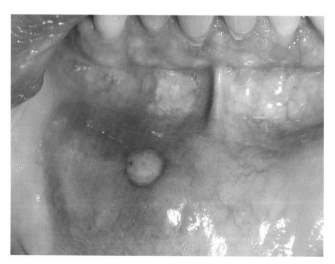

Minor aphthous ulcer on the mandibular labial mucosa

(From Newland JR, *Consultant*, 1989, 29:157-73.)

TREATMENT RECOMMENDATIONS

- Minor ulcers can be palliated with Amlexanox (Aphthasol® *on page 135*)

- Oral lesions may require mild steroid applications including Triamcinolone (Kenalog® *on page 146*) or Fluocinonide (Lidex® ointment *on page 141*)

- Higher potency steroid applications including Dexamethasone (Decadron® *on page 139*) or Clobetasol (Temovate® *on page 138*) are not usually indicated in treatment of these mild forms of ulceration, however, in major aphthae may be required

  - Triamcinolone (Kenalog® in Orabase® 0.1% *on page 146*)

  - 0.05% Fluocinonide (Lidex®) ointment or gel *on page 141*

  - Clobetasol propionate (Temovate® *on page 138*) ointment 0.05% (high potency topical corticosteroid)

  - Dexamethasone (Decadron® elixir 0.5 mg/5 mL *on page 139*)

- To achieve systemic effect if desired, a rinse and swallow regimen can be designed by the clinician. Some clinicians have recommended tapering the dosage after 3 days of q.i.d. swallowing to swallowing only once a day for 3 days and ultimately ending with 3 days of q.i.d. rinsing alone. The potency of dexamethasone usually leads to resolution of the lesion(s) without the need for systemic effect.

- In severe or persistent cases, other immunomodulators, including thalidomide in variable doses, 50-300 mg/day, have shown efficacy.

FOLLOW-UP

- Long-term steroid use should be avoided without medical collaboration

- Periodic biopsy for any malignant changes is appropriate

- Re-evaluate as symptoms change, but at least at each recall

- Select potency based on severity

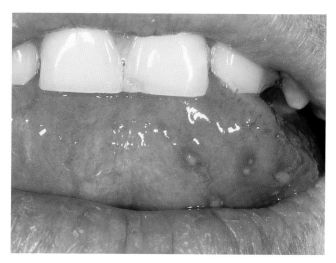

A cluster of herpetiform aphthous ulcers on the ventral tongue

CLINICAL SIGNIFICANCE

- Major aphthous ulcers can heal with scar formation

- Recurrent aphthous ulcers can be a component of Behcet's syndrome (oral mucosal, conjunctival, and genital ulcers)

PRIMARY HERPETIC GINGIVOSTOMATITIS

ETIOLOGY

- Acute infection with herpes simplex virus (usually type 1) in an individual with no previous exposure to the virus (no neutralizing antibodies)

- Virus is spread by direct contact with contaminated saliva

TYPICAL VISUAL CUES

- Multiple vesicles which quickly rupture to form small superficial ulcers

- Small ulcers can merge into larger ulcers

- Any oral mucosal site can be involved (both keratinized and nonkeratinized mucosa

- Gingiva is diffusely enlarged and erythematous (there may be spontaneous bleeding from the gingival sulcus)

- Lesions can also involve perioral skin

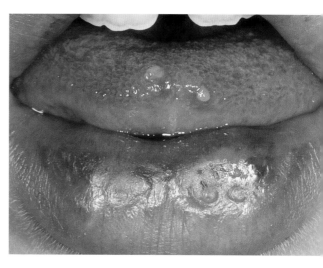

Vesicle and ulcers on the tongue of a child with primary herpetic gingivostomatitis

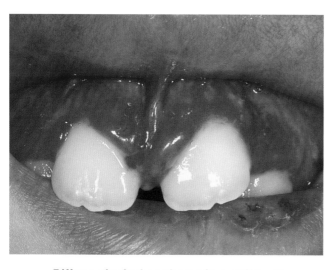

Diffuse gingival erythema in a child with primary herpetic gingivostomatitis

OTHER USEFUL CLINICAL INFORMATION

- Occurs most often in children

- Painful cervical lymphadenopathy can precede the onset of oral lesions

- Fever, difficulty eating, irritability, and malaise often accompany the infection

DIFFERENTIAL DIAGNOSIS

- Aphthous ulcers

- Recurrent intraoral herpes

- Herpes zoster

- Herpangina

- Erythema multiforme

DIAGNOSTIC STEPS

- Definitive diagnosis can usually be made on the basis of clinical presentation

- A cytologic smear can be prepared from the ulcer surface and stained with Papanicolaou stain to demonstrate the presence of virus (viral cytopathic effect)

TREATMENT RECOMMENDATIONS

- Acyclovir oral, 200 mg, 5 times/day *on page 134* or Acyclovir ointment (Zovirax® *on page 134*)

- Other treatments include prevention with Lysine tablets *on page 143*, 500 mg, 2-4 times/day during the period of prodrome

- Applications of Penciclovir (Denavir® *on page 145*) can also give symptomatic relief and improve the speed of healing

- Docosanol (Abreva® *on page 140*), an OTC medication, has also been approved

- These lesions are self-limiting, however, and generally run a course of 7-14 days

- Antibiotic for secondary infection in primary herpetic gingivostomatitis - Pen Vee-K, 500 mg *on page 145*

- Diphenhydramine (Benadryl® elixir *on page 140*) in Kaopectate® 50:50 rinse and expectorate for symptomatic relief prior to meals to help maintain nutrition

CLINICAL SIGNIFICANCE

- In the majority of patients, the primary infection is asymptomatic

- In symptomatic patients, the primary infection typically exhibits a clinical course of one to two weeks, and the oral mucosal lesions usually heal uneventfully

- After the primary infection, herpes simplex virus remains latent in the trigeminal ganglion and can be reactivated to cause recurrent lesions

- Both the vesicular and ulcerated stages of the infection are contagious and can pose an occupational risk for dentists and dental hygienists

- Immunocompromised individuals are at increased risk of contracting a primary infection

RECURRENT HERPES

SYNONYMS

- Fever Blisters
- Cold Sores

ETIOLOGY

- Reactivation of herpes simplex virus (usually type 1)
- Virus leaves the trigeminal ganglion and travels down a branch of the trigeminal nerve to produce recurrent lesions on perioral skin or oral mucosa
- Reactivation of the virus can be triggered by aging, exposure to sunlight, local trauma, physical or emotional stress, and immunosuppression

TYPICAL VISUAL CUES

- Clusters of small blisters (vesicles) which quickly rupture to form small ulcers
- Small ulcers frequently merge to form larger ulcers
- Involvement of the lower lip (recurrent herpes labialis) is the most common manifestation of recurrent herpes
- Lesions often extend to perioral skin and are covered with a hemorrhagic crust
- Intraoral lesions (recurrent intraoral herpes) are less common than recurrent herpes labialis, and tend to occur on keratinized mucosa (attached gingiva and hard palate)

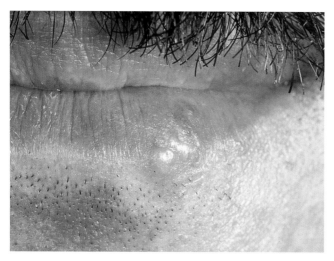

Clustered vesicle of recurrent herpes labialis

OTHER USEFUL CLINICAL INFORMATION

- Recurrent lesions are commonly preceded by a prodrome of itching, burning, or tingling
- The lesions are usually associated with local discomfort
- Multiple recurrences are common

DIFFERENTIAL DIAGNOSIS

- Aphthous ulcers
- Herpes zoster
- Herpangina
- Erythema multiforme
- Necrotizing ulcerative gingivitis
- Ulcers associated with systemic disease

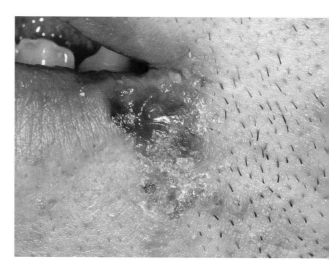

Clustered vesicles and ulcers of recurrent herpes labialis

DIAGNOSTIC STEPS

- A definitive diagnosis can usually be made on the basis of clinical presentation
- A cytologic smear can be prepared from the ulcer surface and stained with Papanicolaou stain to demonstrate the presence of virus (viral cytopathic effect)

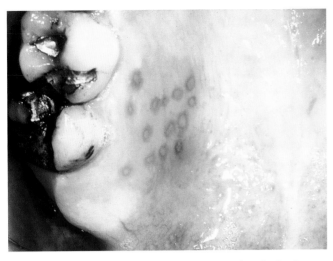

Recurrent intraoral herpes on the palatal gingiva (the ulcers were preceded by vesicles)

(Copyright © *Texas Dental Journal.* Used with permission)

TREATMENT RECOMMENDATIONS

- Acyclovir oral, 200 mg, 5 times/day (Zovirax® *on page 134*) or Acyclovir ointment *on page 134*

- Valacyclovir *on page 146* 2 g twice daily for one day (doses separated by 12 hours)

- Other treatments that include prevention with Lysine tablets (Enisyl® *on page 143*), 500 mg, 2-4 times a day during the period of prodrome

- Applications of Penciclovir (Denavir® *on page 145*) can also give symptomatic relief and improve the speed of healing

- Docosanol (Abreva® *on page 140*), an OTC medication, has also been approved

- These lesions are self-limiting, however, and generally run a course of 7-14 days

- Antibiotic for secondary infection in primary herpetic gingivostomatitis and ANUG
  - Pen Vee-K, 500 mg *on page 145*
  - Acyclovir ointment (Zovirax®) 5% *on page 134*
  - Penciclovir cream (Denavir® *on page 145*)
  - Acyclovir tablets (treatment and prophylaxis) *on page 134*

- Systemic medication for treatment of recurrent herpes simplex OTC
  - Lysine tablets, 500 mg *on page 143*

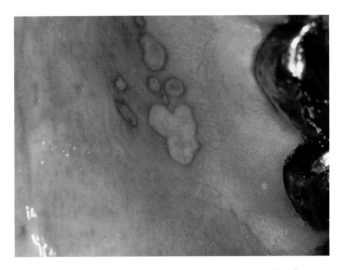

Recurrent intraoral herpes on the palatal gingiva (the ulcers were preceded by vesicles)

(From Newland JR, *Consultant*, 1989, 29:159-73)

CLINICAL SIGNIFICANCE

- Recurrent lesions typically heal uneventfully within 7-10 days

- In immunocompromised individuals, recurrent lesions can be more persistent

- Both the vesicular and ulcerated stages of the infection are contagious and can pose an occupational risk for dentists and dental hygienists

- Recurrent herpes can trigger erythema multiforme

HERPANGINA

ETIOLOGY

- An acute infection caused by various strains of Coxsackie type A virus

- Transmitted by contaminated saliva

TYPICAL VISUAL CUES

- Multiple small blisters (vesicles) that quickly rupture to form small superficial ulcers

- Affected mucosa is erythematous

- Typically located on the soft palate and tonsillar fauces

- Erythematous pharyngitis is also commonly present

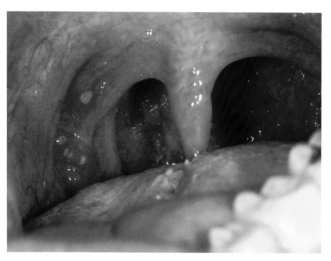

Ulcers of herpangina on the tonsillar fauces

OTHER USEFUL CLINICAL INFORMATION

- Occurs most often in children

- More common during the summer months

- Usually quite painful

- Associated with fever, sore throat, difficulty eating, an malaise

DIFFERENTIAL DIAGNOSIS

- Aphthous ulcers

- Primary herpetic gingivostomatitis

- Recurrent intraoral herpes

- Herpes zoster

DIAGNOSTIC STEPS

- Definitive diagnosis can usually be made on the basi of clinical presentation

- The presence of small ulcers localized to the soft palat and tonsillar fauces is characteristic of herpangina

TREATMENT RECOMMENDATIONS

- Condition is usually self-limiting and treatment include supportive care only

CLINICAL SIGNIFICANCE

- The lesions typically heal within 7-10 days

- Immunity develops to the specific viral strain causin the infection, and the individual will not be infected b that strain again: however, infection can be caused b another strain

HERPES ZOSTER

SYNONYMS

- Shingles

ETIOLOGY

- An acute recurrent infection caused by varicella zoster virus

- The initial infection in an individual with no previous exposure is called varicella zoster (chickenpox)

- Following the initial infection, virus remains latent in sensory ganglia (latent virus in the trigeminal ganglion can cause intraoral lesions)

- Reactivation of the virus can be triggered by local trauma, immunosuppression (cancer chemotherapy, acquired immunodeficiency syndrome), and malignancy (especially leukemia and lymphoma)

TYPICAL VISUAL CUES

- Clusters of small blisters (vesicles) that quickly rupture to form small superficial ulcers

- Occur on both keratinized and nonkeratinized mucosa

- Usually extend to, but do not cross the midline

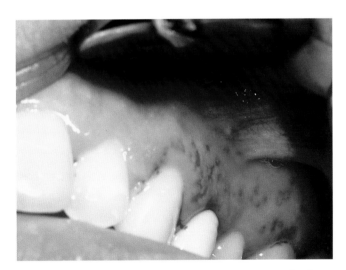

Clustered ulcers of herpes zoster on attached gingiva (the ulcers were preceded by vesicles)

OTHER USEFUL CLINICAL INFORMATION

- Lesions may be preceded by a prodrome of pain and paresthesia

- They are associated with severe pain

DIFFERENTIAL DIAGNOSIS

- Aphthous ulcers
- Primary herpetic gingivostomatitis
- Recurrent intraoral herpes
- Herpangina
- Erythema multiforme

DIAGNOSTIC STEPS

- Definitive diagnosis can usually be made on the basis of clinical presentation

- A cytologic smear can be prepared from the ulcer surface and stained with Papanicolaou stain to demonstrate the presence of virus (viral cytopathic effect)

- A cytologic smear can be stained with fluorescein-labeled monoclonal antibodies to varicella zoster virus to differentiate from herpes simplex virus

TREATMENT RECOMMENDATIONS

- In healthy patients - supportive care only is sufficient; in immunocompromised patients - Acyclovir (Zovirax® *on page 134*), Vidarabine, or Interferon (Intron A® *on page 142*) may be indicated

- Valacyclovir (*on page 146*) 1 g 3 times/day for 7 days

CLINICAL SIGNIFICANCE

- Severe pain caused by post herpetic neuralgia may persist for months after the oral mucosal lesions resolve

- Recurrent episodes of herpes zoster may be associated with undiagnosed malignancy

PRIMARY SYPHILIS

SYNONYMS

- Chancre

ETIOLOGY

- Initial infection with the spirochete *Treponema pallidum*

- Usually transmitted by sexual activity

- Oral mucosal lesions transmitted by urogenital contact

TYPICAL VISUAL CUES

- Indurated deep-seated ulcer with elevated margins

- Occur most often on the lips and tongue (at the site of inoculation)

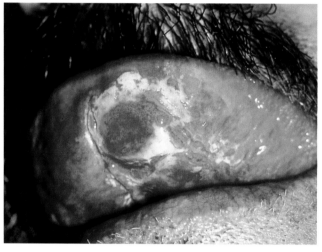

A chancre of primary syphilis on the ventral tongue

OTHER USEFUL CLINICAL INFORMATION

- Develops a few weeks after inoculation

- Characteristically painless

- Cervical lymphadenopathy develops one week after chancre appears

DIFFERENTIAL DIAGNOSIS

- Tuberculosis

- Deep-seated fungal infection

- Large traumatic ulcer

- Squamous cell carcinoma

DIAGNOSTIC STEPS

- Serologic tests for antibodies to *Treponema pallidum* are usually positive within the first few week of infection

- Microscopic examination may be necessary to confirm the diagnosis (biopsy tissue can be treated with special silver stains to demonstrate the presence of *Treponema pallidum*)

TREATMENT RECOMMENDATIONS

- Management is usually by the patient's physician and includes high-dose penicillin

  (See the current edition of Wynn RL, Meiller TF, and Crossley HL, *Drug Information Handbook for Dentistry*, Hudson, OH: Lexi-Comp, Inc, for information on these drugs)

CLINICAL SIGNIFICANCE

- The chancre will heal spontaneously within several weeks, even without treatment; however, some patients are at risk of developing secondary syphilis

- Chancres are contagious and thus pose an occupational risk for members of the dental team

SECONDARY SYPHILIS

SYNONYMS

- Mucous Patches

ETIOLOGY

- Secondary infection with the spirochetes *Treponema pallidum*

TYPICAL VISUAL CUES

- Multiple superficial ulcers covered with a white to yellow pseudomembrane

- Occur most often on the tongue, lips, buccal mucosa, and soft palate

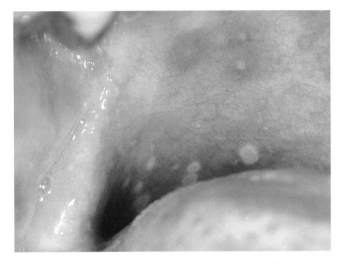

**Mucous patches of secondary syphilis
on the soft palate**

OTHER USEFUL CLINICAL INFORMATION

- Patients often complain of sore throat, fever, weight loss, and malaise

- May exhibit a cutaneous maculopapular rash

DIFFERENTIAL DIAGNOSIS

- Pseudomembranous candidiasis

- Plaque-type lichen planus

DIAGNOSTIC STEPS

- Serologic tests for *Treponema pallidum* are positive during secondary syphilis

- A smear can be prepared from the ulcer surface and stained with specific immunofluorescent antibodies to *Treponema pallidum*

TREATMENT RECOMMENDATIONS

- Management is usually by the patient's physician and includes high-dose penicillin

  (See the current edition of Wynn RL, Meiller TF, and Crossley HL, *Drug Information Handbook for Dentistry*, Hudson, OH: Lexi-Comp, Inc, for information on these drugs)

CLINICAL SIGNIFICANCE

- Mucous patches will heal spontaneously within a few weeks, even without treatment; however, in some individuals, the organisms enter a period of latency (latent syphilis)

- These individuals are at risk of developing tertiary syphilis many years later

- Mucous patches are contagious and thus pose an occupational risk for members of the dental team

TUBERCULOSIS

ETIOLOGY

- An oral mucosal infection caused by *Mycobacterium tuberculosis*

- Oral mucosal lesions secondary to pulmonary tuberculosis

- Pre-existing oral wound (such as an extraction site) inoculated with infected sputum

- Occasionally spread through blood vessels to oral tissues

TYPICAL VISUAL CUES

- Ulcerated granulomatous mass

- Tongue and palate are most common sites

- May involve a recent extraction site

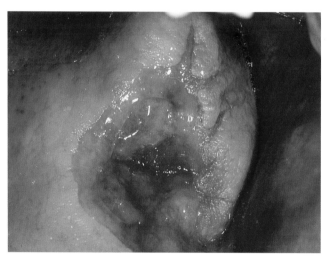

Tuberculosis arising in an extraction site (the patient has pulmonary tuberculosis)

OTHER USEFUL CLINICAL INFORMATION

- Persistent, painful ulceration

- Patient may have a chronic cough

- Patient may describe low-grade fever, night sweats, malaise, weight loss, and chest pain

- More common in urban, poor immigrants (Southeast Asia and the Caribbean) and immunocompromised individuals (especially AIDS patients)

DIFFERENTIAL DIAGNOSIS

- Primary syphilis

- Deep-seated fungal infection

- Traumatic ulcerative granuloma

- Squamous cell carcinoma

- Wegener's granulomatosis

DIAGNOSTIC STEPS

- Refer for tuberculin skin test

- Refer for chest radiograph

- Microscopic examination is necessary to confirm the diagnosis (biopsy reveals granulomas with caseous necrosis and multinucleated giant cells (tubercle)

- Acid-fast bacillus (AFB) stain demonstrates infective organisms

TREATMENT RECOMMENDATIONS

- Management is usually by the patient's physician and may include isoniazid, rifampin, streptomycin, or ethambutol often given in combination

  (See the current edition of Wynn RL, Meiller TF, and Crossley HL, *Drug Information Handbook for Dentistry*, Hudson, OH: Lexi-Comp, Inc, for information on these drugs)

CLINICAL SIGNIFICANCE

- Oral mucosal lesions are contagious and thus pose an occupational risk for dental hygienists and dentists

- Relapse following treatment suggests immunocompromised status

- Infection may be resistant to usual chemotherapy (multidrug resistant tuberculosis)

- Infection may present as a submandibular mass (submandibular lymph node infected with tuberculosis is called scrofula)

DEEP FUNGAL INFECTION / HISTOPLASMOSIS

ETIOLOGY

- An infection caused by inhalation of fungal spores

- Infective organisms include *Histoplasma capsulatum* (histoplasmosis), *Coccidioides immitis* (coccidioidomycosis), *Blastomyces dermatitidis* (blastomycosis), and *Cryptococcus neoformans* (cryptococcosis)

- Oral lesions secondary to pulmonary infection

- Pre-existing wound (such as an extraction site) inoculated with infected sputum

- Occasionally spread through blood vessels to oral tissues

TYPICAL VISUAL CUES

- Ulcerated granulomatous mass

- Tongue, palate, and gingiva most common sites

- May involve a recent extraction site

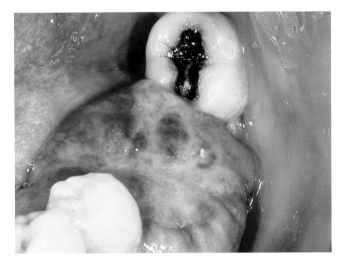

Histoplasmosis arising in an extraction site (the patient has pulmonary histoplasmosis)

OTHER USEFUL CLINICAL INFORMATION

- Persistent, painful ulceration

- Patient may have a chronic cough

- Patient may describe low-grade fever, night sweats, malaise, and weight loss

DIFFERENTIAL DIAGNOSIS

- Primary syphilis

- Tuberculosis

- Traumatic ulcerative granuloma

- Squamous cell carcinoma

- Wegener's granulomatosis

DIAGNOSTIC STEPS

- Refer for serologic testing

- Refer for chest radiograph

- Microscopic examination necessary to confirm diagnosis (biopsy reveals granulomatous proliferation with multinucleated giant cells; staining with periodic acid-Schiff (PAS) stain or Grocott-Gomori methenamine silver (GMS) stain will demonstrate the organisms)

TREATMENT RECOMMENDATIONS

- Management is usually by the patient's physician and may include Amphotericin B (Fungizone® *on page 136*) or Ketoconazole (Nizoral® *on page 142*)

CLINICAL SIGNIFICANCE

- Oral mucosal lesions are contagious and thus may pose an occupational risk to dental hygienists and dentists

- Relapse following treatment suggests immunocompromised status

WEGENER'S GRANULOMATOSIS

ETIOLOGY

- An inflammatory disease characterized by necrotizing granulomas involving the upper and lower respiratory tract and kidneys

- The precise etiology is unknown; however, it may be the result of immunologic dysfunction

TYPICAL VISUAL CUES

- Deep granulomatous ulcers involving the palate

- Focal erythematous gingival swelling with a pebbly, strawberry-like surface (strawberry gingivitis)

- May cause destruction of alveolar bone with subsequent tooth mobility

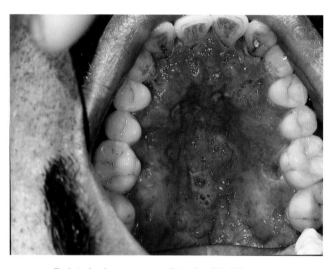

Palatal ulcers associated with Wegener's granulomatosis

OTHER USEFUL CLINICAL INFORMATION

- More common in adults

- Lesions may also be present in lungs and kidneys

DIFFERENTIAL DIAGNOSIS

- Tuberculosis

- Deep fungal infection

- Necrotizing sialometaplasia

- Squamous cell carcinoma

- Salivary gland carcinoma

DIAGNOSTIC STEPS

- Definitive diagnosis requires the correlation of clinical presentation of the disease with the microscopic features of a granulomatous lesion

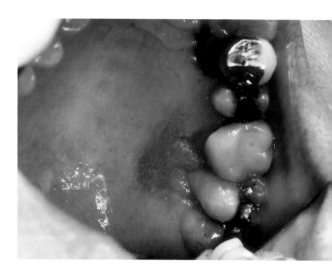

Strawberry gingivitis associated with Wegener's granulomatosis

TREATMENT RECOMMENDATIONS

- Treatment supervised by the patient's physician may include systemic prednisone combined with immunosuppressive agents such as Cyclophosphamide (on page 139) and Methotrexate (on page 143)

FOLLOW-UP

- Careful clinical follow-up is essential

CLINICAL SIGNIFICANCE

- Oral mucosal lesions may be the first indication of disease

NECROTIZING ULCERATIVE GINGIVITIS

SYNONYMS

- NUG

- Trench Mouth

- Vincent's Infection

ETIOLOGY

- An acute infection caused by fusospirochetal bacteria (*Fusobacterium nucleatum* and spirochetes including *Borrelia vencentii* and *Prevotella intermedia*)

- Predisposing factors include physical and emotional stress, local trauma, poor nutrition, poor oral hygiene, and compromised immune status

TYPICAL VISUAL CUES

- Crateriform ulcerations of the interdental papillae

- Necrosis may extend to adjacent gingival tissues

- Spontaneous gingival hemorrhage

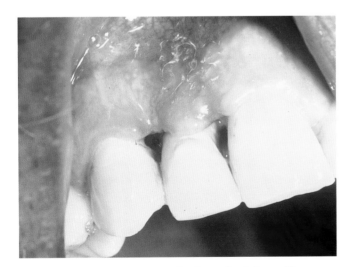

Craterform ulcers on the interdental papillae in necrotizing ulcerative gingivitis

OTHER USEFUL CLINICAL INFORMATION

- More common in young adult males

- Ulcers usually associated with severe pain and fetid odor

- Patients often complain of fever and malaise

- Swollen, tender, cervical lymph nodes may be present

DIFFERENTIAL DIAGNOSIS

- Primary herpetic gingivostomatitis

- Aphthous ulcers

- Erosive lichen planus

- Cicatricial pemphigoid

- Erythema multiforme

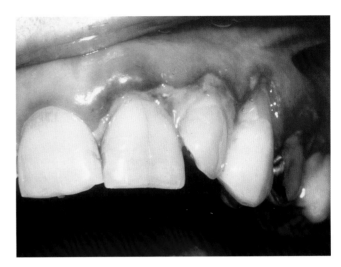

Gingival ulcers in necrotizing ulcerative gingivitis

DIAGNOSTIC STEPS

- Definitive diagnosis can usually be made on the basis of clinical presentation

- No diagnostic steps beyond recognition of clinical features

TREATMENT RECOMMENDATIONS

- Treatment includes debridement (multiple visits), anti-microbial mouthrinse (Listerine® *on page 136*), and chlorhexidine rinses *on page 138*. Patient may need antibiotic support with Metronidazole (Flagyl® *on page 144*) and/or Penicillin (*on page 145*)

CLINICAL SIGNIFICANCE

- Can progress to acute necrotizing ulcerative stomatitis in immunocompromised patients (especially HIV-infected individuals)

NECROTIZING SIALOMETAPLASIA

ETIOLOGY

- Loss of blood supply to minor salivary gland tissue with resulting ischemic necrosis

TYPICAL VISUAL CUES

- Deep-seated ulcer preceded by erythematous swelling
- Typically located on the hard palate off the midline

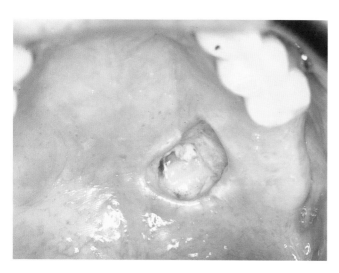

Necrotizing sialometaplasia on the hard palate

OTHER USEFUL CLINICAL INFORMATION

- More common in adult males
- Often associated with pain or paresthesia

DIFFERENTIAL DIAGNOSIS

- Primary syphilis
- Tuberculosis
- Deep-seated fungal infection
- Squamous cell carcinoma
- Salivary gland carcinoma
- Wegener's granulomatosis

DIAGNOSTIC STEPS

- Microscopic examination necessary to confirm diagnosis

TREATMENT RECOMMENDATIONS

- Once a diagnosis is confirmed, no intervention is necessary
- Lesion usually heals within two months

CLINICAL SIGNIFICANCE

- Can mimic malignancy both clinically and microscopically
- Careful evaluation essential to avoid inaccurate diagnosis and inappropriate treatment

ULCERS ASSOCIATED WITH SYSTEMIC DISEASE

ETIOLOGY

- Diminished immunologic function with increased susceptibility to bacterial infection

- Infection commonly occurs at site of previous traumatic injury or periodontal infection

- Specific predisposing conditions include blood dyscrasia such as cyclic neutropenia and agranulocytosis, immunologic disorders such as Crohn's disease, and cancer chemotherapy

TYPICAL VISUAL CUES

- Ulcers, usually superficial, with an erythematous border

- Occasionally, more deep-seated

- Occur most often on buccal mucosa, labial mucosa, tongue, and gingiva

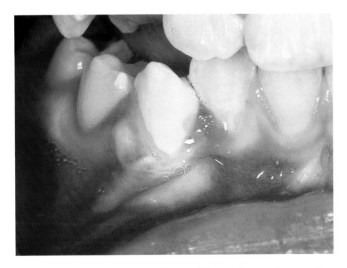

A gingival ulcer in a patient with cyclic neutropenia

OTHER USEFUL CLINICAL INFORMATION

- Ulcers are usually chronic and painful

- They may exhibit multiple recurrences

- Patient may exhibit other manifestations of underlying systemic disease (fever, malaise, and weight loss)

DIFFERENTIAL DIAGNOSIS

- Aphthous ulcers

- Traumatic ulcers

- Necrotizing ulcerative gingivitis

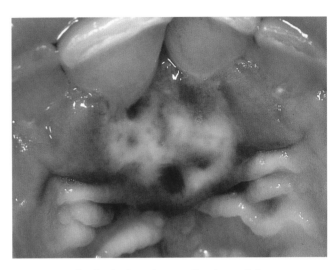

A gingival ulcer in a patient receiving chemotherapy for leukemia

DIAGNOSTIC STEPS

- Diagnosis can usually be made on the basis of history and clonal presentation

- If systemic disease is suspected and there is no positive history, patient should be referred for appropriate medical evaluation

TREATMENT RECOMMENDATIONS

- Palliation of oral ulcers

- Treat underlying systemic disease

CLINICAL SIGNIFICANCE

- Oral ulcerations may be first indication of underlying systemic disease

SQUAMOUS CELL CARCINOMA

ETIOLOGY

- Squamous epithelial origin

- Precise etiology unknown

- Risk factors include tobacco, alcohol, solar radiation (lower lip), genetic predisposition, nutritional deficiency (iron-deficiency anemia in Plummer-Vinson syndrome), immunosuppression, and infections (candidal leukoplakia and human papillomavirus infections)

TYPICAL VISUAL CUES

- Deep-seated ulcerated mass (extending into the adjacent tissues)

- Fungating ulcerated mass (extending away from the adjacent tissues)

- Ulcer margins commonly elevated

- Adjacent tissues commonly firm to palpation (indurated)

- May be residual leukoplakia and/or erythroplakia

- Occurs most often on posterior lateral tongue, oropharynx, and floor of the mouth

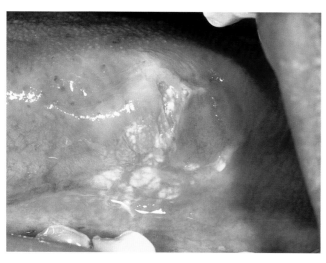

Squamous cell carcinoma on the posterior lateral tongue

(From Newland JR, "Oral Ulcers," *Difficult Diagnosis 2*, Taylor RB (ed), Philadelphia, PA: WB Saunders, 1992)

OTHER USEFUL CLINICAL INFORMATION

- Continuous enlargement

- More common in adult males

- Positive cervical lymphadenopathy may be present

- Local pain, referred pain (often to the ear), and paresthesia (often of the lower lip)

DIFFERENTIAL DIAGNOSIS

- Primary syphilis

- Tuberculosis

- Deep fungal infection

- Traumatic ulcerated granuloma

- Wegener's granulomatosis

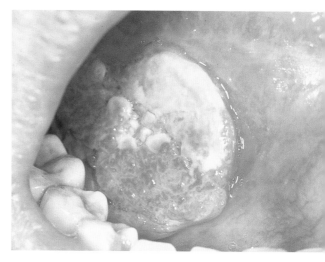

Squamous cell carcinoma on the posterior lateral tongue

(From Newland JR, *Consultant*, 1989, 29:159-73)

DIAGNOSTIC STEPS

- Routine cytologic smear or brush biopsy can be performed from the ulcer surface; however, microscopic examination of biopsy tissue is necessary to confirm the diagnosis

TREATMENT RECOMMENDATIONS

- Patient should be counseled to stop smoking

- Appropriate combination of surgery, radiation therapy, and chemotherapy where indicated

- Careful periodic re-evaluation

CLINICAL SIGNIFICANCE

- Early diagnosis is essential for cure

- Presence of lymph node metastasis greatly worsens the prognosis

- Approximately 50% of patients have evidence of lymph node metastasis at time of diagnosis

- Patients who have had one oral cancer are at greater risk of having a second oral cancer

SALIVARY GLAND CARCINOMA

ETIOLOGY

- Adenocarcinomas of minor salivary gland origin

- Precise etiology is unknown

TYPICAL VISUAL CUES

- Deep-seated ulcerated mass

- Lesion surface may exhibit telangiectatic blood vessels

- Occur most often on the hard palate off the midline

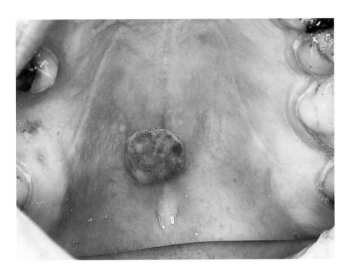

Salivary gland cancer on the hard palate

OTHER USEFUL CLINICAL INFORMATION

- Continuous enlargement

- More common in adults

- Often associated with local discomfort

- May exhibit evidence of bone destruction on radiographs

DIFFERENTIAL DIAGNOSIS

- Primary syphilis

- Tuberculosis

- Deep-seated fungal infection

- Benign salivary gland neoplasm (especially early cancers)

- Necrotizing sialometaplasia

- Wegener's granulomatosis

DIAGNOSTIC STEPS

- Microscopic examination is necessary to confirm the diagnosis

TREATMENT RECOMMENDATIONS

- Appropriate surgery and radiation therapy

- Careful periodic re-evaluation

CLINICAL SIGNIFICANCE

- Palate is the most common site for minor salivary gland neoplasms

- Approximately half of these are malignant

- Local recurrence following treatment is common

- Metastasize most often to lungs and bone

BLISTERING / SLOUGHING LESIONS

GENERAL PRINCIPLES

- Oral mucosal blisters can result from extrinsic injury (mucosal burns), or from intrinsic causes (commonly associated with an immunologic defect such as an allergic reaction or an autoimmune disease).

- The blisters associated with these diseases are usually larger than half a centimeter in diameter so they qualify as bulla (in contrast to smaller blisters called vesicles which are more often a manifestation of viral infection).

- Blister formation results from damage to some component of the oral mucosa causing separation of the tissue either within the epithelium (an intraepithelial blister), or at the epithelial-connective tissue interface (a subepithelial blister).

- When a blister ruptures, the surface sloughs (patients often notice sloughing of gingival tissues when they are brushing their teeth).

- Sloughing can also occur in the absence of blister formation.

- Once the blister ruptures and the surface sloughs, the lesion becomes ulcerated.

- Blistering/sloughing lesions are usually associated with severe local discomfort.

- When localized to gingiva, the term desquamative gingivitis can be used to describe these lesions.

- The presence of these diseases on gingiva can interfere with proper oral hygiene and predispose to plaque-related gingival disease.

LIST OF DISEASES

Erosive / Bullous Lichen Planus ... 74
Cicatricial Pemphigoid ... 76
Pemphigus Vulgaris ... 78
Paraneoplastic Pemphigus ... 80
Mucosal Burns ... 81
Erythema Multiforme ... 82
Lupus Erythematosus ... 84

EROSIVE / BULLOUS LICHEN PLANUS

ETIOLOGY

- A defect in cell-mediated immunity resulting in damage to the basal cells of oral epithelium

- This causes epithelial sloughing in erosive lichen planus and subepithelial blister formation in bullous lichen planus

TYPICAL VISUAL CUES

- Erosive lichen planus appears clinically as mucosal erosions that can slough to form superficial ulcerations

- Bullous lichen planus presents as blisters that quickly rupture to form superficial ulcerations

- Keratotic striations and/or plaques may or may not be present

- Erosive/bullous lichen planus occurs most often on the posterior buccal mucosa and adjacent mandibular buccal vestibule

- Lesions may also involve the tongue, gingiva, and labial mucosa

- Gingival lesions produce desquamative gingivitis

- When on gingiva, plaque-related gingivitis may also be present because it is too painful for the patient to brush effectively

OTHER USEFUL CLINICAL INFORMATION

- Occurs with greatest frequency in middle-aged women

- Commonly associated with local discomfort ranging from a burning sensation to severe pain

DIFFERENTIAL DIAGNOSIS

- Cicatricial pemphigoid (especially for gingival lesions)

- Pemphigus vulgaris (especially for gingival lesions)

- Paraneoplastic pemphigus

- Erythema multiforme

- Lupus erythematosus

- Mucosal burns

DIAGNOSTIC STEPS

- Incisional biopsy should be performed with half the tissue placed in formalin for routine histopathologic examination and half in Michel's solution for direct immunofluorescent studies

- Direct immunofluorescent studies may be necessary to differentiate erosive/bullous lichen planus from cicatricial pemphigoid and pemphigus vulgaris (in lichen planus, direct immunofluorescence reveals deposits of fibrinogen along the epithelial basement membrane zone)

Erosive lichen planus on the attached gingiva

(From Newland JR, "Oral Ulcers," *Difficult Diagnoses 2*, Taylor RB (ed), Philadelphia, PA: WB Saunders, 1992)

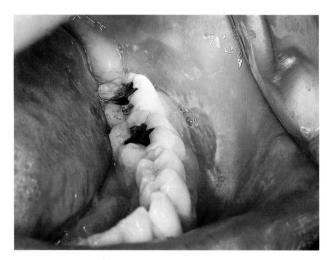

Bullous lichen planus on the buccal mucosa

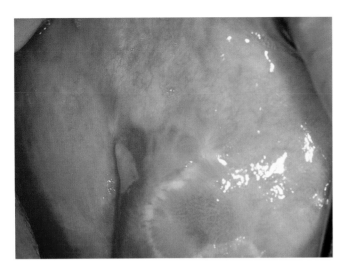

Erosive lichen planus on the buccal mucosa; the erosions are encircled with adherent white striations

TREATMENT RECOMMENDATIONS

- Oral lesions may require mild steroid applications including Triamcinolone (Kenalog® in Orabase® *on page 146*) or Fluocinonide (Lidex® ointment *on page 141*)

- Higher potency steroid applications including Dexamethasone (Decadron® *on page 139*) or Clobetasol (Temovate® *on page 138*) are not usually indicated in treatment of mild forms of lichen planus

- Benzocaine (Orabase® with Benzocaine *on page 137*) for extremely mild cases

- Triamcinolone (Kenalog® in Orabase® *on page 146*) 0.1% for mild cases

- 0.05% Fluocinonide (Lidex® ointment or gel *on page 141*)

- Dexamethasone (Decadron® *on page 139*) elixir 0.5 mg/5 mL

- Clobetasol propionate (Temovate® *on page 138*) ointment 0.05% (high-potency topical corticosteroid)

- To achieve systemic effect, if desired, a rinse and swallow regimen can be designed by the clinician. Some clinicians have recommended tapering the dosage after 3 days of q.i.d. swallowing to swallowing only once a day for 3 days and ultimately ending with 3 days of q.i.d. rinsing alone. The potency of dexamethasone usually leads to resolution of the lesion(s) without the need for systemic effect.

- During severe episodes, prescribing systemic steroids, such as Prednisone *(on page 145)* or Methylprednisolone *(on page 143)* possibly coupled with immunomodulators, such as Azathioprine *(on page 136)*, Cyclophosphamide *(on page 139)*, Tacrolimus *(on page 146)*, Dapsone *(on page 139)*, Cyclosporine *(on page 139)*, or Methotrexate *(on page 143)* may be considered in close collaboration with the patient's physician.

FOLLOW-UP

- Patients with lichen planus need reassurance that these lesions need to be observed, but that they are not likely to be premalignant

- This does not, however, preclude regular follow-up, biopsy, if appropriate, and observation

- Symptomatic management of the lichenoid areas including topical steroids such as Triamcinolone (Kenalog® *on page 146*) or Fluocinonide (Lidex® *on page 141*)

- More potent steroids including Clobetasol (Temovate® *on page 138*) or Dexamethasone (Decadron® *on page 139*) may be indicated based on symptomatology

- Long-term steroid use should be avoided without medical collaboration

- Periodic biopsy for any malignant changes is appropriate

- Re-evaluate as symptoms change, but at least at each recall

CLINICAL SIGNIFICANCE

- Lesions of erosive/bullous lichen planus are sometimes secondarily infected with *Candida albicans*

- In women, vaginal mucosal lesions may accompany the oral mucosal lesions

- Allergic mucosal reactions which resemble lichen planus can develop following the use of certain systemic medications (lichenoid drug reactions)

- Mucosal reactions to dental amalgam can also resemble lichen planus (contact lichenoid reactions)

CICATRICIAL PEMPHIGOID

SYNONYMS

- Benign Mucous Membrane Pemphigoid

ETIOLOGY

- A defect in cell-mediated immunity resulting in damage to the epithelial basement membrane

- This causes the epithelium to separate from the underlying connective tissue (subepithelial blister formation)

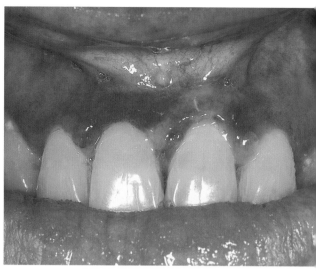

Desquamative gingivitis caused by cicatricial pemphigoid

TYPICAL VISUAL CUES

- Blisters which rupture to cause desquamation and ulceration

- Can involve any oral mucosal site; however, gingiva is the most common location (desquamative gingivitis)

- When on gingiva, plaque-related gingivitis may also be present because it is often too painful for the patient to brush effectively

OTHER USEFUL CLINICAL INFORMATION

- Occurs with greatest frequency in middle-aged women

- Commonly associated with severe pain

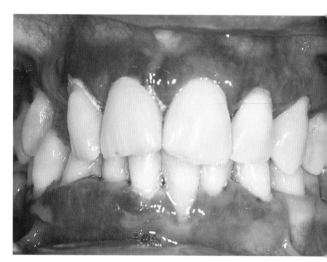

Desquamative gingivitis caused by cicatricial pemphigoid

DIFFERENTIAL DIAGNOSIS

- Erosive/bullous lichen planus (especially for gingival lesions)

- Pemphigus vulgaris (especially for gingival lesions)

- Paraneoplastic pemphigus

- Erythema multiforme

- Lupus erythematosus

DIAGNOSTIC STEPS

- Incisional biopsy should be performed with half the tissue placed in formalin for routine histopathologic examination and half in Michel's solution for direct immunofluorescent studies

- Direct immunofluorescent studies may be necessary to differentiate cicatricial pemphigoid from erosive/bullous lichen planus and pemphigus vulgaris (in cicatricial pemphigoid, direct immunofluorescence reveals deposits of IgG and compliment C3 along the epithelial basement membrane zone)

TREATMENT RECOMMENDATIONS

- Oral lesions may require mild steroid applications including Triamcinolone (Kenalog® *on page 146*) or Fluocinonide (Lidex® ointment *on page 141*)

- Higher potency steroid applications including Dexamethasone (Decadron® *on page 139*) or Clobetasol (Temovate® *on page 138*) may be indicated in treatment of pemphigoid and pemphigus

- Systemic steroids, such as Prednisone *(on page 145)* or Methylprednisolone (Medrol® dose packs *on page 143*) may be indicated in collaboration with the patient's physician

- During severe episodes, prescribing systemic steroids, such as Prednisone *(on page 145)* or Methylprednisolone *(on page 143)* possibly coupled with immunomodulators, such as Azathioprine *(on page 136)*, Cyclophosphamide *(on page 139)*, Tacrolimus *(on page 146)*, Dapsone *(on page 139)*, Cyclosporine *(on page 139)*, or Methotrexate *(on page 143)* may be considered in close collaboration with the patient's physician.

FOLLOW-UP

- Long-term steroid use should be avoided without medical collaboration

- Periodic biopsy for any malignant changes is appropriate

- Re-evaluate as symptoms change, but at least at each recall

CLINICAL SIGNIFICANCE

- Other possible sites of involvement include conjunctiva, larynx, vaginal mucosa in women, and skin (skin lesions are uncommon)

- Conjunctival scarring associated with cicatricial pemphigoid can be a cause of blindness

PEMPHIGUS VULGARIS

ETIOLOGY

- An immunologic defect that causes the production of autoantibodies against desmosomes which hold adjacent epithelial cells together

- Destruction of desmosomes causes adjacent epithelial cells to separate (acantholysis) producing an intraepithelial blister

TYPICAL VISUAL CUES

- Blisters which rupture to form erosions and ulcerations

- Any oral mucosal site can be involved

- Gingival lesions produce desquamative gingivitis

- When on gingiva, plaque-related gingivitis may also be present because it is often too painful for the patient to brush effectively

OTHER USEFUL CLINICAL INFORMATION

- Occurs with equal frequency in men and women, and is more common in people of Jewish descent

- Associated with severe discomfort

- Patients may exhibit a positive Nikolsky sign (the formation of a blister on apparently normal skin after slight mechanical pressure)

DIFFERENTIAL DIAGNOSIS

- Erosive/bullous lichen planus (especially for gingival lesions)

- Cicatricial pemphigoid (especially for gingival lesions)

- Paraneoplastic pemphigus

- Erythema multiforme

- Lupus erythematosus

DIAGNOSTIC STEPS

- Incisional biopsy should be performed with half the tissue placed in formalin for routine histopathologic examination and half in Michel's solution for direct immunofluorescent studies

- Direct immunofluorescent studies may be necessary to differentiate pemphigus vulgaris form erosive/bullous lichen planus and cicatricial pemphigoid (in pemphigus vulgaris, direct immunofluorescence reveals the presence of IgG and compliment C3 in the intercellular spaces between adjacent epithelial cells)

- Autoantibodies can be demonstrated in patients' serum by indirect immunofluorescence

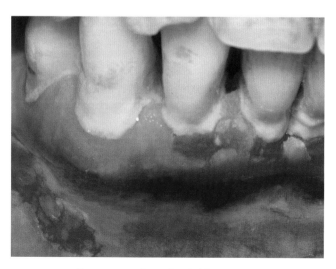

**Desquamative gingivitis caused
by pemphigus vulgaris**

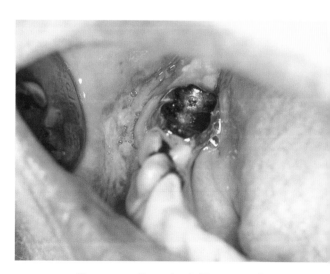

**Desquamative gingivitis caused
by pemphigus vulgaris**

TREATMENT RECOMMENDATIONS

- Oral lesions are seldom treated in isolation from systemic disease

- Steroids are the treatment of choice when working with the physician; Prednisone (*on page 145*) is often employed in combination with steroid-sparing drugs such as Azathioprine (Imuran® *on page 136*)

- Management of the oral lesions of pemphigus vulgaris can include applications of the same topical corticosteroids used in the treatment of pemphigoid

- During severe episodes, prescribing systemic steroids, such as Prednisone (*on page 145*) or Methylprednisolone (*on page 143*) possibly coupled with immunomodulators, such as Azathioprine (*on page 136*), Cyclophosphamide (*on page 139*), Tacrolimus (*on page 146*), Dapsone (*on page 139*), Cyclosporine (*on page 139*), or Methotrexate (*on page 143*) may be considered in close collaboration with the patient's physician.

CLINICAL SIGNIFICANCE

- Skin lesions of pemphigus vulgaris are potentially life-threatening

- Approximately 50% of patients with pemphigus vulgaris present with oral mucosal lesions before the onset of skin lesions

- Lesions resembling pemphigus (paraneoplastic pemphigus) can occur in patients with leukemia and lymphoma

PARANEOPLASTIC PEMPHIGUS

SYNONYMS

- Neoplasia-Induced Pemphigus

ETIOLOGY

- Occurs most often in patients with leukemia or lymphoma

- Cross-reaction between neoplasia-related antibodies and oral mucosal antigens causes epithelial damage with blister formation

TYPICAL VISUAL CUES

- Blisters which rupture to form erosions and ulcerations

- Any oral mucosal site can be involved

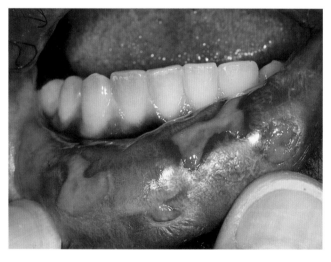

Ruptured blister associated with paraneoplastic pemphigus on the lower lip

OTHER USEFUL CLINICAL INFORMATION

- More common in adults

- The oral mucosal lesions are painful

- Similar lesions can develop on skin, conjunctiva, and vaginal mucosa

DIFFERENTIAL DIAGNOSIS

- Erosive/bullous lichen planus
- Pemphigus vulgaris
- Cicatricial pemphigoid
- Erythema multiforme

DIAGNOSTIC STEPS

- Definitive diagnosis requires correlation of clinical presentation with a history of leukemia or lymphoma

- Microscopically, paraneoplastic pemphigus can resemble erosive/bullous lichen planus, cicatricial pemphigoid, or pemphigus vulgaris

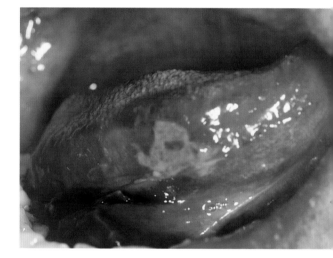

Ruptured blisters associated with paraneoplastic pemphigus on the tongue

TREATMENT RECOMMENDATIONS

- Treatment supervised by the patient's physician may include systemic prednisone combined with immuno-suppressive agents such as Cyclophosphamide (*or page 139*) and Methotrexate (*on page 143*)

FOLLOW-UP

- Careful clinical follow-up essential

CLINICAL SIGNIFICANCE

- Aggressive treatment of the paraneoplastic pemphigus may exacerbate the underlying malignancy

MUCOSAL BURNS

ETIOLOGY

- Thermal injury from hot foods (especially those heated in a microwave oven)

- Chemical burns from aspirin and other chemical (silver nitrate, phenol, and endodontic medicaments)

TYPICAL VISUAL CUES

- Desquamation of the involved mucosa with superficial ulceration

- Most commonly affect the palate (food-related burns), gingiva (aspirin burns), and buccal/labial mucosa (burns from endodontic medicaments)

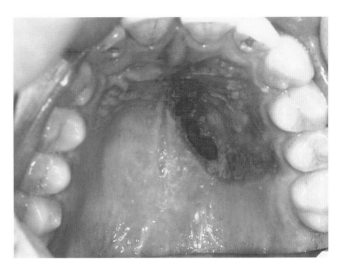

Mucosal burn caused by hot pizza cheese

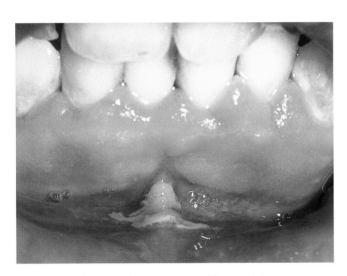

Mucosal burn caused by aspirin

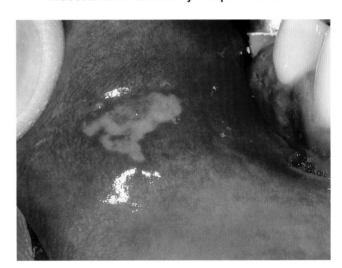

Mucosal burn caused by an endodontic medicament

OTHER USEFUL CLINICAL INFORMATION

- Patients usually report a history of thermal or chemical injury

- Mucosal burns are commonly associated with severe local discomfort

DIFFERENTIAL DIAGNOSIS

- Because of the clinical history, mucosal burns are infrequently confused with other blistering/sloughing lesions included in this section

DIAGNOSTIC STEPS

- Definitive diagnosis can usually be made on the basis of patient history and clinical presentation

- No other diagnostic steps are necessary

TREATMENT RECOMMENDATIONS

- Generally, intraoral burns heal without complication; however, topical steroids such as Triamcinolone (Kenalog® in Orabase® *on page 146*) or Fluocinonide (Lidex® *on page 141*) may be helpful

- Secondary infection may occur and require antibiotics such as Penicillin V Potassium (*on page 145*) or Clindamycin (*on page 138*)

- Antimicrobial mouthrinses, such as Listerine® (*on page 136*) or Chlorhexidine (Peridex®, Periogard® *on page 138*) can reduce or prevent this secondary infection

ERYTHEMA MULTIFORME

ETIOLOGY

- For half the patients with erythema multiforme, the precise cause is unknown

- In the other half, an immunologic defect (perhaps an allergic/hypersensitivity reaction) is thought to be the cause

- The hypersensitivity reaction can be triggered by a preceding infection (usually viral or fungal) or by exposure to various medications (most commonly analgesics and antibiotics)

TYPICAL VISUAL CUES

- Multiple blisters, erosions, and ulcerations affecting virtually any oral mucosal site

- Hemorrhagic crusting at the vermilion of the lips is a characteristic feature

OTHER USEFUL CLINICAL INFORMATION

- Exhibits an acute onset

- More common in young adult males

- Erythematous skin lesions (target lesions) may occur on skin (especially of the extremities)

DIFFERENTIAL DIAGNOSIS

- Primary herpetic gingivostomatitis

- Major aphthous ulcers

- Erosive/bullous lichen planus

- Cicatricial pemphigoid

- Pemphigus vulgaris

- Paraneoplastic pemphigus

DIAGNOSTIC STEPS

- If the disease has an acute onset and the characteristi lesions (hemorrhagic crusting of the vermilion of the lip and target lesions on skin) are present, the diagnosi can usually be made on the basis of clinical presenta tion

- A cytologic smear can be performed to rule out herpeti infection

- A biopsy can be performed to rule out erosive/bullou lichen planus, cicatricial pemphigoid, and pemphigu vulgaris

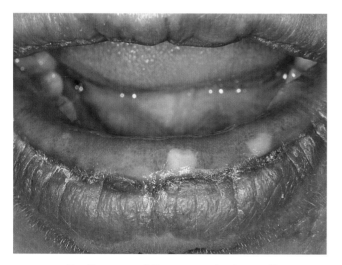

Erythema multiforme on the lower lip
(note the characteristic hemorrhagic crusting along the vermilion border)

(Copyright © *Texas Dental Journal.* Used with permission)

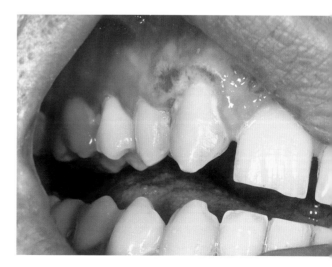

Desquamative gingivitis caused by erythema multiforme

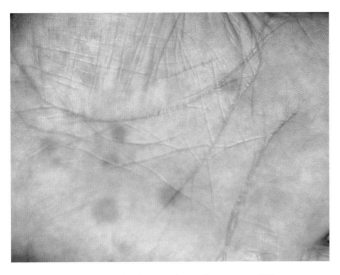

**Typical target lesions of erythema multiforme
on the palmar skin**

(Copyright © *Texas Dental Journal.* Used with permission)

TREATMENT RECOMMENDATIONS

- Systemic steroids in collaboration with the physician managing the case; however, there is some controversy regarding systemic steroids in EM

- Also, Acyclovir (*on page 134*) 800-1200 mg/day in 2-3 divided doses may be useful if EM is triggered by HSV

- Valacyclovir (*on page 146*) 500 mg/day

CLINICAL SIGNIFICANCE

- Stevens-Johnson syndrome is a more severe manifestation of erythema multiforme characterized by oral mucosal lesions, skin lesions, conjunctival lesions, and genital lesions

- Steven's Johnson syndrome is a potentially life-threatening disease

LUPUS ERYTHEMATOSUS
(Chronic Cutaneous, Subacute Cutaneous, Systemic)

ETIOLOGY

- An autoimmune disease involving defects in both the humoral and cellular immune systems

- Circulating and tissue-bound autoantibodies have been identified to a variety of cellular components

- It is speculated that a genetic defect or viral infection may trigger the autoimmune reaction

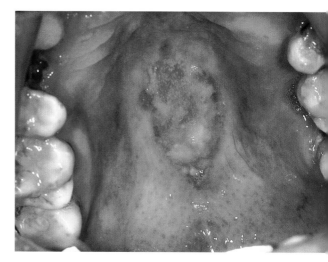

Lupus erythematosus on the mucosa of the hard palate

TYPICAL VISUAL CUES

- Areas of erythema, erosion, and superficial ulceration frequently associated with keratosis striations (can closely resemble the oral mucosal lesions of erosive lichen planus)

- Most common intraoral sites of involvement are buccal mucosa, gingiva, and lip

OTHER USEFUL CLINICAL INFORMATION

- Occurs more commonly in young to middle-aged women

- Scaly erythematous patches localized to sun-exposed skin (butterfly rash involving the malar areas and bridge of the nose)

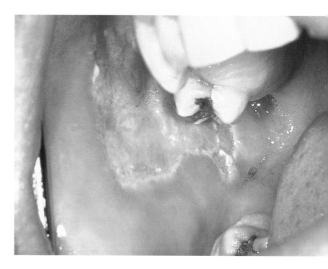

Lupus erythematosus on the buccal mucosa

DIFFERENTIAL DIAGNOSIS

- Erosive lichen planus

- Cicatricial pemphigoid

- Pemphigus vulgaris

- Erythema multiforme

- Mucosal allergy

DIAGNOSTIC STEPS

- Incisional biopsy should be performed with half the tissue placed in formalin for routine histopathologic examination and half in Michel's solution for direct immunofluorescent studies

- Direct immunofluorescent studies may be necessary to differentiate lupus erythematosus from erosive lichen planus, cicatricial pemphigoid, and pemphigus vulgaris (in lupus erythematosus, direct immunofluorescence reveals shaggy deposits of IgM, IgG, and compliment C3 along the epithelial basement membrane zone)

TREATMENT RECOMMENDATIONS

- Topical steroids, such as Fluocinonide (Lidex® *on page 141*) for DLE; systemic steroids in collaboration with the patient's physician for SLE

- Oral lesions may require mild steroid applications including Triamcinolone (Kenalog® *on page 146*) or Fluocinonide (Lidex® ointment *on page 141*)

- Higher potency steroid applications including Dexamethasone (Decadron® *on page 139*) or Clobetasol (Temovate® *on page 138*) may be indicated in treatment of mild forms of DLE

- For systemic LE, systemic steroids are usually indicated and drugs such as Dapsone (*on page 139*) have shown some efficacy

CLINICAL SIGNIFICANCE

- Patients with chronic cutaneous lupus erythematosus only have skin and mucosal lesions

- In subacute cutaneous lupus erythematosus, patients may have rheumatoid arthritis and musculoskeletal diseases in addition to skin and mucosal lesions

- Potentially life-threatening involvement of the kidneys and heart can occur in systemic lupus erythematosus

PIGMENTED LESIONS

GENERAL PRINCIPLES

- Pigmented lesions can result from external sources of pigment such as amalgam, or from internal sources such as melanin or red blood cells.

- Multiple oral mucosal pigmentations can be associated with systemic disease (Addison's disease for example).

- The primary concern when evaluating pigmented oral mucosal lesions is to exclude malignancies such as malignant melanoma and Kaposi's sarcoma.

LIST OF DISEASES

Physiologic Pigmentation 88
Amalgam Tattoo 89
Black Hairy Tongue 90
Melanotic Macule 91
Peutz-Jegher's Syndrome 92
Addison's Disease 93
Smokers Melanosis 94
Melanocytic Nevus 95
Kaposi's Sarcoma 96
Malignant Melanoma 98

PHYSIOLOGIC PIGMENTATION

ETIOLOGY

- Pigmentation caused by normal amounts of melanin in basal cells of oral epithelium

TYPICAL VISUAL CUES

- Diffuse tan to brown pigmentation

- Located most often on the attached gingiva

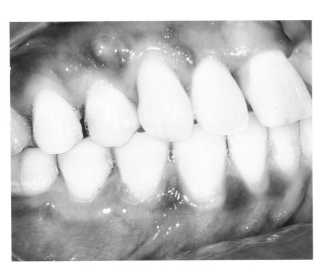

Physiologic gingival pigment

OTHER USEFUL CLINICAL INFORMATION

- Painless

- Persistent

- Occurs most often in individuals with dark skin

DIFFERENTIAL DIAGNOSIS

- Because of its characteristic clinical appearance, physiologic pigmentation is infrequently confused with other pigmented lesions included in this section

DIAGNOSTIC STEPS

- A definitive diagnosis can usually be made on the basis of clinical presentation

- No diagnostic steps beyond recognition of clinical features

TREATMENT RECOMMENDATIONS

- No treatment necessary

AMALGAM TATTOO

SYNONYMS

- Focal Argyrosis

ETIOLOGY

- Contamination of a pre-existing oral mucosal wound with amalgam particles
- Usually secondary to dental restorative treatment or apical surgery

TYPICAL VISUAL CUES

- Circumscribed darkly pigmented (gray to black) macule
- Overlying mucosa is intact
- Occur most often on gingiva and adjacent mucosa

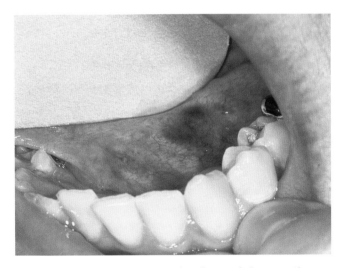

An amalgam tattoo on the floor of the mouth

OTHER USEFUL CLINICAL INFORMATION

- Painless
- Persistent
- History of previous dental treatment involving the use of amalgam
- Amalgam particles occasionally visible on radiographs

DIFFERENTIAL DIAGNOSIS

- Melanotic macule
- Melanocytic nevus
- Malignant melanoma

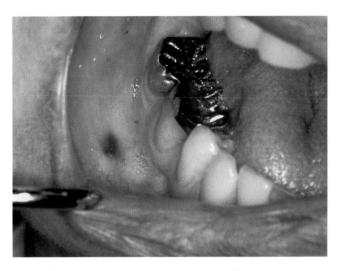

An amalgam tattoo on the buccal mucosa

DIAGNOSTIC STEPS

- Clinical evidence of previous amalgam restorations in the area
- A definitive diagnosis can usually be made on the basis of clinical presentation
- Microscopic examination is indicated if diagnosis can not be made on clinical presentation alone

TREATMENT RECOMMENDATIONS

- No treatment necessary once diagnosis is confirmed

CLINICAL SIGNIFICANCE

- If there is any doubt about the diagnosis based on clinical features, a biopsy is essential to exclude the possibility of malignant melanoma

BLACK HAIRY TONGUE

ETIOLOGY

- Formation of excess keratin causes elongation of the filiform papillae on the dorsal tongue

- The keratin becomes pigmented by pigment-producing bacteria and/or components in tobacco, beverages (especially coffee and tea), and foods

- May be infected with *Candida albicans*

TYPICAL VISUAL CUES

- Elongation of the filiform papillae

- Brown to black pigmentation

- Located on the posterior dorsal tongue

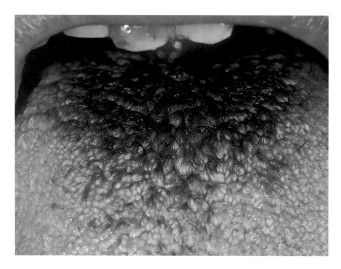

Black Hairy Tongue

OTHER USEFUL CLINICAL INFORMATION

- Patients often have poor oral hygiene

- May complain of a bad taste

DIFFERENTIAL DIAGNOSIS

- Because of its characteristic clinical appearance, black hairy tongue is infrequently confused with other pigmented lesions included in this section

DIAGNOSTIC STEPS

- Definitive diagnosis can usually be made on the basis of clinical presentation

- No diagnostic steps beyond recognition of clinical features

- Cytology smear with PAS to rule out fungal involvement

TREATMENT RECOMMENDATIONS

- Elimination of predisposing factors

- Cleaning the dorsal tongue with a soft toothbrush

- Treat candidiasis, if present, as in pseudomembranous *Candida* infections

CLINICAL SIGNIFICANCE

- Despite similar names, should not be confused with the HIV-related lesion hairy leukoplakia

MELANOTIC MACULE

SYNONYMS

- Focal Melanosis

ETIOLOGY

- Solar radiation (lower lip lesions)
- Etiology of oral mucosal lesions unknown

TYPICAL VISUAL CUES

- A circumscribed tan to brown macule covered with intact mucosa
- Usually less than 0.5 cm in diameter
- Occur most often on lower lip (*labial melanotic macule*) followed by the gingiva, palate, and buccal mucosa (*oral melanotic macule*)

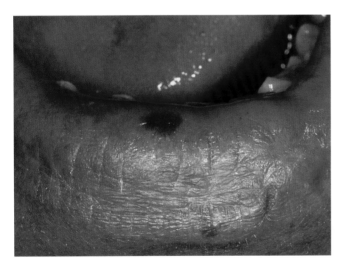

A solitary melanotic macule on the lower lip

OTHER USEFUL CLINICAL INFORMATION

- Painless
- Persistent

DIFFERENTIAL DIAGNOSIS

- Amalgam tattoo
- Melanocytic nevus
- Malignant melanoma

DIAGNOSTIC STEPS

- Microscopic examination necessary to confirm the diagnosis and exclude malignant melanoma (excisional biopsy is likely to remove entire lesion)

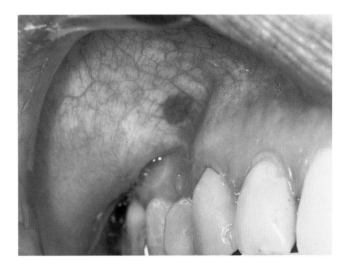

A solitary melanotic macule on the buccal mucosa

TREATMENT RECOMMENDATIONS

- No treatment necessary once diagnosis is confirmed

CLINICAL SIGNIFICANCE

- Multiple labial and oral melanotic macules can be a component of Peutz-Jeghers syndrome and Addison's disease (primary adrenal cortical insufficiency)

PEUTZ-JEGHER'S SYNDROME

ETIOLOGY

- Inherited as an autosomal dominant genetic defect

- Major components of the syndrome are mucocutaneous melanotic macules and intestinal polyps

TYPICAL VISUAL CUES

- Multiple, circumscribed, tan to brown macules covered with intact mucosa

- Occur most often on labial mucosa and buccal mucosa

- Occasionally occur on tongue and palate

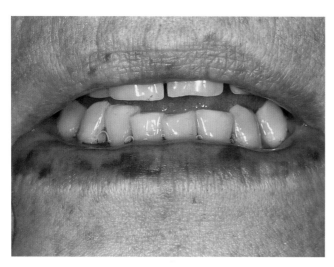

Melanotic macules of Peutz-Jegher's syndrome on the lower lip

OTHER USEFUL CLINICAL INFORMATION

- Melanotic macules commonly involve skin around the mouth

- May also involve skin around the nose and anus, as well as skin on the palms of the hands and soles of the feet

- Patients may have a history of bowel obstruction caused by the intestinal polyps

DIFFERENTIAL DIAGNOSIS

- Because of the characteristic clinical presentation (mucocutaneous melanotic macules and patient history of intestinal polyps), Peutz-Jegher's syndrome is infrequently confused with other pigmented lesions included in this section

- In the absence of typical patient history, Addison's disease should be included in the differential diagnosis

DIAGNOSTIC STEPS

- A definitive diagnosis can usually be made on the basis of clinical presentation and patient history

- No diagnostic steps beyond recognition of clinical features

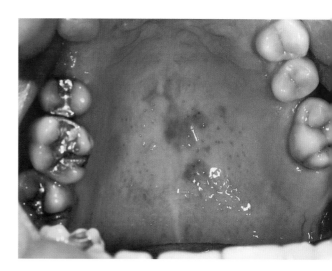

Melanotic macules of Peutz-Jegher's syndrome on the hard palate

TREATMENT RECOMMENDATIONS

- No treatment necessary for oral mucosal macules

FOLLOW-UP

- Patient should be carefully followed by appropriate physicians

CLINICAL SIGNIFICANCE

- Intestinal polyps can cause bowel obstruction

- Increased incidence of cancers involving the intestines, pancreas, genital tract, and breast

ADDISON'S DISEASE

SYNONYMS

- Adrenal Cortical Insufficiency

ETIOLOGY

- Destruction of the adrenal gland cortex caused by auto-immune disease, infection, or metastatic cancer

- Loss of adrenocortical hormones causes increased production of ACTH which stimulates melanocytes

TYPICAL VISUAL CUES

- Multiple, circumscribed, dark brown to black macules covered with intact mucosa

- Any oral mucosal site can be involved

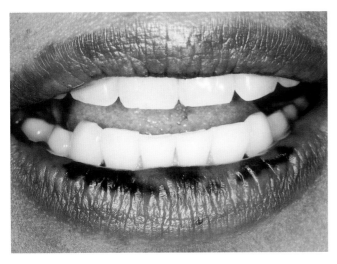

Melanotic macules of Addison's disease on the lower lip

OTHER USEFUL CLINICAL INFORMATION

- Generalized brown pigmentation of sun-exposed skin (bronzing of the skin)

- Patients complain of anorexia, nausea, vomiting, fatigue, irritability, depression, weakness, and hypotension

DIFFERENTIAL DIAGNOSIS

- Because of the characteristic clinical presentation (mucosal melanotic macules, bronzing of the skin, and patient history), Addison's disease is infrequently confused with other pigmented lesions included in this section

- In the absence of characteristic clinical presentation, Peutz-Jegher's syndrome should be included in the differential diagnosis

DIAGNOSTIC STEPS

- Definitive diagnosis can usually be made on the basis of clinical presentation and patient history

- Elevated levels of plasma ACTH confirm the diagnosis

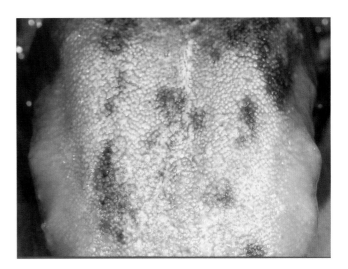

Melanotic macules of Addison's disease on the dorsal tongue

TREATMENT RECOMMENDATIONS

- No treatment necessary for oral mucosal macules

- Corticosteroid replacement therapy supervised by appropriate physicians

FOLLOW-UP

- Patients should be followed by appropriate physicians

CLINICAL SIGNIFICANCE

- Oral mucosal lesions are frequently the first indication of disease

- Stress associated with dental treatment may require increased dose of corticosteroid

SMOKERS MELANOSIS

SYNONYMS

- Smoking-Associated Melanosis

ETIOLOGY

- Irritants in tobacco smoke stimulate melanocytes to synthesize excess melanin

- Female sex hormones, especially those in oral contraceptives, appear to be a predisposing factor

TYPICAL VISUAL CUES

- Diffuse, irregular, dark brown macules

- Covered with intact mucosa

- Located most often on anterior labial mucosa (cigarette smoking), buccal mucosa, and palate (pipe smoking)

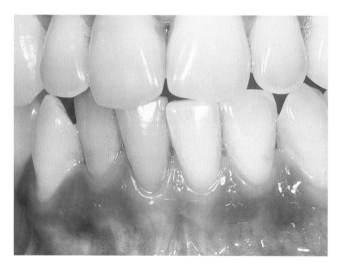

Smokers melanosis on the mandibular labial gingiva

OTHER USEFUL CLINICAL INFORMATION

- More common in women who smoke and use oral contraceptives

DIFFERENTIAL DIAGNOSIS

- Multiple oral melanotic macules

- Physiologic pigmentation

DIAGNOSTIC STEPS

- Documentation of a smoking history and oral contraceptive use in women

- Definitive diagnosis can usually be made on the basis of clinical presentation

TREATMENT RECOMMENDATIONS

- Patient should be counseled to stop smoking

- Lesions will then usually resolve within several months to a few years

CLINICAL SIGNIFICANCE

- Smokers melanosis does not appear to be a premalignant lesion

- No treatment necessary

MELANOCYTIC NEVUS

ETIOLOGY

- A benign neoplasm of melanin-producing cells (melanocytes)
- Can be either congenital (present at birth) or acquired (arising later in life)

TYPICAL VISUAL CUES

- Circumscribed, tan to brown, papular lesion
- Usually less than 0.5 cm in diameter
- Covered with intact mucosa
- Located most often on the hard palate

DIFFERENTIAL DIAGNOSIS

- Amalgam tattoo
- Melanotic macule
- Malignant melanoma

DIAGNOSTIC STEPS

- Microscopic examination is necessary to confirm the diagnosis and to exclude malignant melanoma

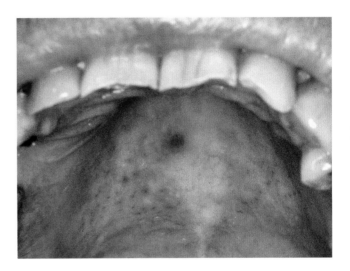

Melanocytic nevus on the hard palate

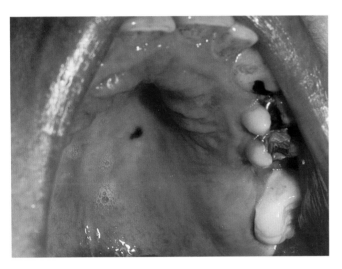

Melanocytic nevus on the hard palate

OTHER USEFUL CLINICAL INFORMATION

- Painless
- Persistent
- More common in women

TREATMENT RECOMMENDATIONS

- No treatment necessary once the diagnosis has been confirmed

CLINICAL SIGNIFICANCE

- Nevi with microscopic evidence of junctional activity may develop into malignant melanoma

KAPOSI'S SARCOMA

ETIOLOGY

- A malignancy of blood vessels

- Cytomegalovirus has been implicated as a possible cause

- Loss of immunologic surveillance increases the risk for Kaposi's sarcoma (a component of acquired immuno-deficiency syndrome)

DIFFERENTIAL DIAGNOSIS

- Hematoma

- Hemangioma

- Pyogenic granuloma

- Malignant melanoma

TYPICAL VISUAL CUES

- Bluish-purple macule, plaque, or nodule

- The surface is usually intact

- Located most often on hard palate and gingiva

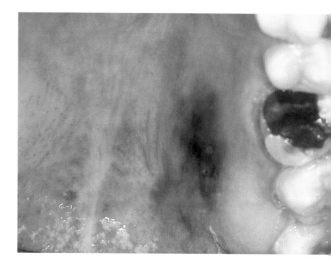

Nodular Kaposi's sarcoma on the palatal gingiva

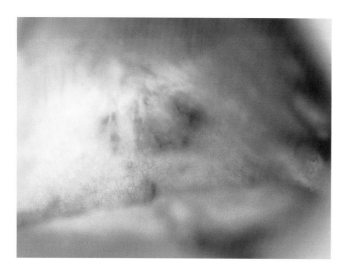

Macular Kaposi's sarcoma on the soft palate

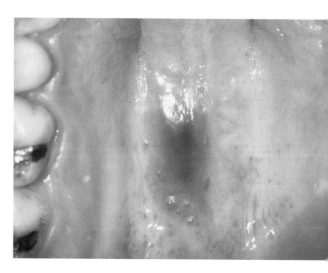

Nodular Kaposi's sarcoma on the hard palate

OTHER USEFUL CLINICAL INFORMATION

- Usually painless

- Continuous enlargement

- More common in young adult males

- The patient will usually have a history of human immu-nodeficiency virus (HIV) infection

- Skin lesions may also be present

DIAGNOSTIC STEPS

- Microscopic examination is necessary to confirm the diagnosis

TREATMENT RECOMMENDATIONS

- Appropriate surgery and chemotherapy

- Determined by symptoms, cosmetic concerns, and staging based on tumor bulk, CD4 count, and "B symptoms"

- Local: Radiotherapy; intralesional vinblastine, surgical excision, cryotherapy, or laser ablation (cosmetic purposes only)

- Systemic: Cytotoxic chemotherapy with various combinations of vincristine, vinblastine, doxorubicin, anthracyclines, etoposide, bleomycin, paclitaxel, and liposomal anthracyclines

- Experimental: Angiogenesis inhibitors, growth factors, cytokine inhibitors, retinoic acids, anti-HHV-8 agents

CLINICAL SIGNIFICANCE

- Kaposi's sarcoma is the most common malignancy associated with AIDS

- More than 50% of patients with Kaposi's sarcoma have oral mucosal lesions

- Oral mucosal Kaposi's sarcoma may be the first manifestation of AIDS

MALIGNANT MELANOMA

ETIOLOGY

- A malignant neoplasm of melanin-producing cells (melanocytes)

- May arise directly from melanocytes in the area of or from a pre-existing nevus (especially those with microscopic evidence of junctional activity)

- Chronic exposure to solar radiation and a fair complexion increases the risk for skin lesions

TYPICAL VISUAL CUES

- Larger than 0.5 cm in diameter

- Irregular margins

- Irregular pigmentation

- Any change in pigmentation

- Ulceration of the overlying mucosa

- Macular (superficial spreading) or elevated (nodular)

- Occurs most often on gingiva and palate

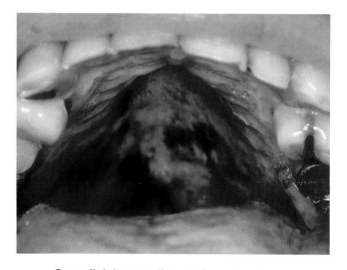

Superficial spreading malignant melanoma on the hard palate

OTHER USEFUL CLINICAL INFORMATION

- Usually painless

- Rapidly enlarging

- Occurs most often in adult males

DIFFERENTIAL DIAGNOSIS

- Amalgam tattoo

- Melanotic macule

- Melanocytic nevus

DIAGNOSTIC STEPS

- Microscopic examination is necessary to confirm the diagnosis

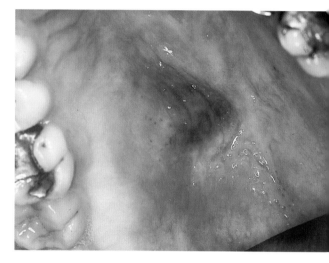

Nodular malignant melanoma on the hard palate

TREATMENT RECOMMENDATIONS

- Appropriate surgery and chemotherapy; refer to appropriate oncology team for aggressive therapy

CLINICAL SIGNIFICANCE

- Malignant melanoma is an extremely aggressive form of cancer

- Early diagnosis is essential for cure

- Patients with oral mucosal lesions generally have a poor prognosis

PAPILLARY LESIONS

GENERAL PRINCIPLES

- When an oral mucosal lesion exhibits a papillary configuration, it suggests that it originated from the squamous epithelial surface.

- Because they are of epithelial origin, the papillary projections are typically white in color because of limited vascularity and/or because of excess keratin (keratin looks white in the mouth).

- Papillary lesions are commonly associated with an infection caused by human papillomavirus.

- The term verrucous (wart-like) is used to describe the surface of papillary lesions when the papillary projections mimic the surface configuration of a cutaneous wart.

LIST OF DISEASES

Squamous Papilloma 100
Verruca Vulgaris 101
Verruciform Xanthoma 102
Condyloma Acuminatum 103
Focal Epithelial Hyperplasia 104
Inflammatory Papillary Hyperplasia 105
Proliferative Verrucous Leukoplakia 106
Verrucous Carcinoma 107

SQUAMOUS PAPILLOMA

ETIOLOGY

- Local trauma

- Human papillomavirus

TYPICAL VISUAL CUES

- Usually a solitary, white, papillary lesion attached with a narrow (pedunculated) base

- Occur most often on the soft palate and ventral tongue

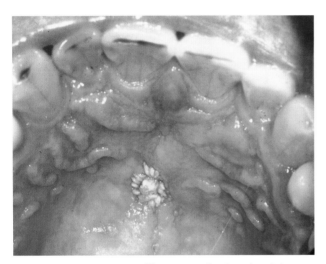

A squamous papilloma on the hard palate

OTHER USEFUL CLINICAL INFORMATION

- Painless

- Persistent

DIFFERENTIAL DIAGNOSIS

- Verruca vulgaris

- Verruciform xanthoma

- Focal epithelial hyperplasia

- Condyloma acuminatum

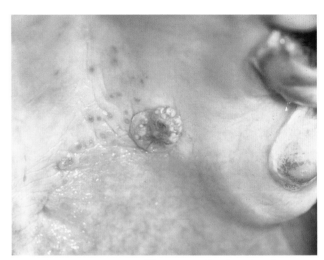

A squamous papilloma on the hard palate

DIAGNOSTIC STEPS

- Microscopic examination necessary to establish a definitive diagnosis

TREATMENT RECOMMENDATIONS

- Local excision

CLINICAL SIGNIFICANCE

- Recurrence is common often due to inadequate excision or viral etiology

VERRUCA VULGARIS

SYNONYMS

- Common Wart

ETIOLOGY

- An infection caused by human papillomavirus (HPV-2, HPV-4, and HPV-40)

TYPICAL VISUAL CUES

- Usually a solitary, white, papillary lesion attached with a narrow (pedunculated) or broad (sessile) base
- Occurs most often on labial mucosa and tongue

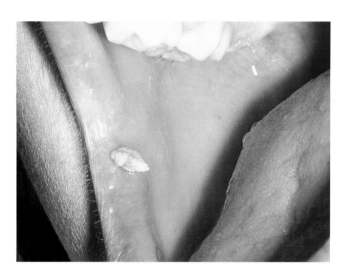

A verruca vulgaris on the lower lip

OTHER USEFUL CLINICAL INFORMATION

- Painless
- Persistent

DIFFERENTIAL DIAGNOSIS

- Squamous papilloma
- Verruciform xanthoma
- Focal epithelial hyperplasia
- Condyloma acuminatum

DIAGNOSTIC STEPS

- Microscopic examination necessary to establish a definitive diagnosis

TREATMENT RECOMMENDATIONS

- Local excision

CLINICAL SIGNIFICANCE

- Lesions may recur following conservative surgical therapy

VERRUCIFORM XANTHOMA

ETIOLOGY

- Precise etiology unknown

- May represent an atypical response to epithelial trauma

TYPICAL VISUAL CUES

- A solitary, white to tan, papillary lesion attached with a broad (sessile) base

- Occurs most often on attached mucosa (attached gingiva and hard palate)

DIFFERENTIAL DIAGNOSIS

- Squamous papilloma

- Verruca vulgaris

- Focal epithelial hyperplasia

- Condyloma acuminatum

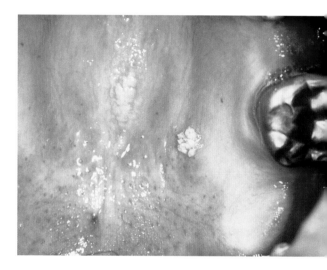

Verruciform xanthoma on the hard palate

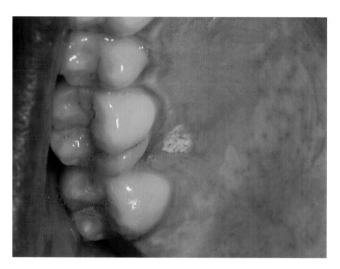

Verruciform xanthoma on the palatal gingiva

DIAGNOSTIC STEPS

- Microscopic examination necessary to establish a definitive diagnosis

OTHER USEFUL CLINICAL INFORMATION

- Painless

- Persistent

- More common in adult females

TREATMENT RECOMMENDATIONS

- Local excision

CLINICAL SIGNIFICANCE

- Recurrence following local excision is uncommon

CONDYLOMA ACUMINATUM

SYNONYMS

- Venereal Wart

ETIOLOGY

- An infection caused by human papillomavirus (HPV-6, HPV-11, HPV-16, and HPV-18)

- A sexually transmitted disease (STD)

TYPICAL VISUAL CUES

- Multiple, pink, slightly papillary nodules attached with broad (sessile) bases

- Commonly arranged in clusters

- Occur most often on lips, tongue, and soft palate

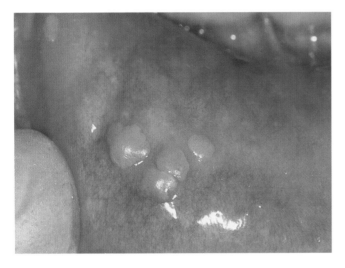

Clustered condyloma acuminata on the lower lip

OTHER USEFUL CLINICAL INFORMATION

- Painless

- Persistent

- More common in young adults

- Anogenital lesions may also be present

DIFFERENTIAL DIAGNOSIS

- Squamous papilloma

- Verruca vulgaris

- Verruciform xanthoma

- Focal epithelial hyperplasia

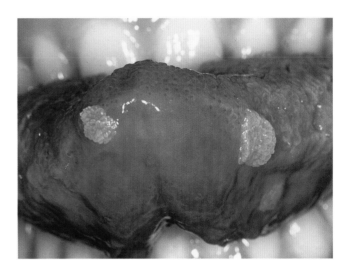

Condyloma acuminata on the tongue

(Copyright © *Texas Dental Journal*. Used with permission)

DIAGNOSTIC STEPS

- Microscopic examination necessary to establish a definitive diagnosis

- Identification of virus by immunohistochemical studies or *in situ* DNA hybridization

TREATMENT RECOMMENDATIONS

- Local excision

- Laser ablation/stripping is commonly used although there is some concern over vaporization of viral particles

CLINICAL SIGNIFICANCE

- Lesions commonly recur following surgical excision

- Reinoculation among sexual partners is common

FOCAL EPITHELIAL HYPERPLASIA

SYNONYMS

- Heck's Disease

ETIOLOGY

- An infection caused by human papillomavirus (HPV-13)

TYPICAL VISUAL CUES

- Multiple, pink, slightly papillary nodules attached with broad (sessile) bases
- Commonly arranged in clusters
- Occur most often on lips, buccal mucosa, and tongue

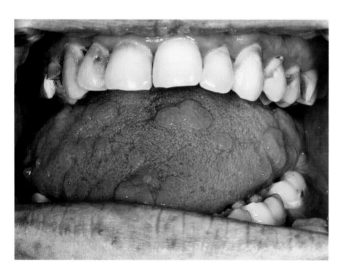

Multiple papillary nodules on the tongue of a patient with focal epithelial hyperplasia

OTHER USEFUL CLINICAL INFORMATION

- Painless
- Persistent
- More common in children and young adults
- May be present in multiple family members

DIFFERENTIAL DIAGNOSIS

- Squamous papilloma
- Verruca vulgaris
- Verruciform xanthoma
- Condyloma acuminatum

DIAGNOSTIC STEPS

- Microscopic examination necessary to establish a definitive diagnosis
- Identification of virus by immunohistochemical studies or *in situ* DNA hybridization

TREATMENT RECOMMENDATIONS

- Local excision
- Lesions often regress spontaneously

INFLAMMATORY PAPILLARY HYPERPLASIA

SYNONYMS

- Palatal Papillomatosis

ETIOLOGY

- Chronic mechanical irritation from an ill-fitting maxillary denture

- Often infected with *Candida albicans*

TYPICAL VISUAL CUES

- Multiple, erythematous, sessile (broad-based) nodules

- Most often located on the mucosa of the palatal vault, occasionally on the alveolar ridge

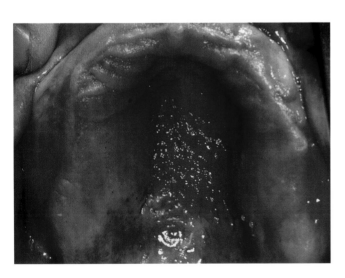

Inflammatory papillary hyperplasia on denture-bearing mucosa of the palatal vault

OTHER USEFUL CLINICAL INFORMATION

- Painless

- Persistent

- More common in older individuals who wear a complete or partial maxillary denture

- Patients often wear dentures continuously (do not remove them at night)

DIFFERENTIAL DIAGNOSIS

- Because of their characteristic clinical appearance, inflammatory papillary hyperplasia is infrequently confused with other papillary lesions included in this section

DIAGNOSTIC STEPS

- No other diagnostic steps other than recognition of characteristic clinical features

- If fungus is considered, cytology smear with PAS is appropriate

TREATMENT RECOMMENDATIONS

- Reline or remake denture

- Treat candidiasis if present. See management of chronic erythematous fungal infection with Nystatin (Mycostatin® *on page 144)*, Clotrimazole (Mycelex® *on page 138)*, or systemic antifungals, Ketoconazole (Nizoral® *on page 142)* or Fluconazole (Diflucan® *on page 140).*

- Remove lesions if they persist (conventional surgery, cryosurgery, electrosurgery, or laser ablation)

CLINICAL SIGNIFICANCE

- Inflammatory papillary hyperplasia often associated with chronic erythematous candidiasis (denture stomatitis)

PROLIFERATIVE VERRUCOUS LEUKOPLAKIA

ETIOLOGY

- Precise etiology unknown
- Often associated with tobacco exposure

TYPICAL VISUAL CUES

- Diffuse, white, papillary or corrugated thickenings
- Commonly involve the tongue and floor of the mouth

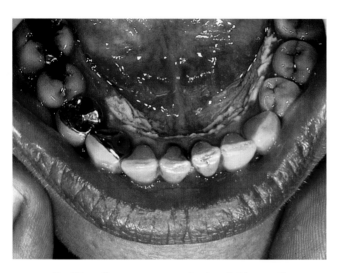

Proliferative verrucous leukoplakia on the floor of the mouth

OTHER USEFUL CLINICAL INFORMATION

- Painless
- Persistent
- More common in women

DIFFERENTIAL DIAGNOSIS

- Verrucous carcinoma

DIAGNOSTIC STEPS

- Microscopic examination is necessary to confirm diagnosis

TREATMENT RECOMMENDATIONS

- Surgical excision, laser ablation is often used
- Periodic re-evaluation

CLINICAL SIGNIFICANCE

- Can eventually develop into verrucous carcinoma conventional squamous cell carcinoma

VERRUCOUS CARCINOMA

SYNONYMS

- Snuff Dipper's Cancer

ETIOLOGY

- Precise cause unknown

- Smokeless tobacco is a significant risk factor

- Human papillomavirus (HPV-16 and HPV-18) has been identified in some lesions

TYPICAL VISUAL CUES

- Diffuse, white, papillary or corrugated thickenings

- Commonly occur on the mandibular buccal vestibule and gingiva (at the site of chronic tobacco exposure)

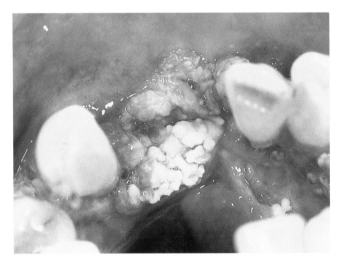

Verrucous carcinoma on the gingiva

OTHER USEFUL CLINICAL INFORMATION

- Painless

- Continuous enlargement

- More common in elderly males

DIFFERENTIAL DIAGNOSIS

- Proliferative verrucous leukoplakia

DIAGNOSTIC STEPS

- Microscopic examination is necessary to confirm the diagnosis

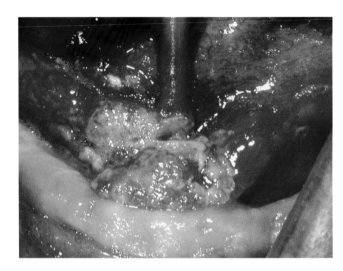

Verrucous carcinoma on the floor of the mouth

TREATMENT RECOMMENDATIONS

- The patient should be counseled to stop using tobacco

- Complete surgical ablation (laser ablation has become popular)

- Periodic re-evaluation

CLINICAL SIGNIFICANCE

- Verrucous carcinomas rarely metastasize, but local recurrence is common

- Conventional squamous cell carcinoma may develop in a pre-existing verrucous carcinoma

SOFT TISSUE ENLARGEMENTS

GENERAL PRINCIPLES

- Soft tissue swellings can be caused by infection, reactive proliferations, and neoplasia.

- Soft tissue swellings arise in the submucosa and usually have sessile (broad) bases.

- The surface of the mass can be smooth, hyperkeratotic (calloused), or ulcerated.

- Because they share some clinical features, it can occasionally be difficult to differentiate between reactive proliferations and malignant neoplasms.

- Multiple oral mucosal soft tissue swellings can be associated with various syndromes, and may be the first indication of the syndrome.

- One or more components of the syndrome may be life-threatening.

LIST OF DISEASES

Pyogenic Granuloma 110
Peripheral Giant Cell Granuloma 111
Peripheral Ossifying Fibroma 112
Fibroma 113
Epulis Fissuratum 114
Mucocele 115
Ranula 116
Parulis 117
Actinomycosis 118
Lipoma 119
Hemangioma 120
Lymphangioma 121
Neuroma 122
Neurofibroma 123
Lymphoid Hyperplasia 124
Oral Lymphoepithelial Cyst 125
Gingival Cyst of the Adult 126
Cheilitis Glandularis 127
Benign Salivary Gland Neoplasms 128
Drug-Induced Gingival Hyperplasia 129
Leukemic Gingival Infiltrate 130
Metastatic Carcinoma 131

PYOGENIC GRANULOMA

SYNONYMS

- Pregnancy Tumor (localized lesion)
- Pregnancy Gingivitis (generalized lesions)

ETIOLOGY

- A reactive hyperplasia of vascularized granulation tissue that develops in response to local irritating factors (bacterial plaque and/or calculus)
- Hormonal changes associated with pregnancy are a contributing factor for gingival lesions (pregnancy tumor)

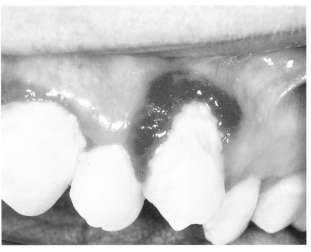

A pyogenic granuloma on the gingiva

TYPICAL VISUAL CUES

- A solitary, circumscribed, red nodule attached with a broad (sessile) or narrow (pedunculated) base
- The surface can be lobulated and is commonly ulcerated
- The lesion may bleed spontaneously or on gentle manipulation
- More than 75% occur on gingiva (less frequently on labial mucosa, tongue, or buccal mucosa)

OTHER USEFUL CLINICAL INFORMATION

- Firm to palpation
- Usually painless
- Persistent (chronic)
- More common in women
- Commonly associated with pregnancy
- Gingival lesions associated with poor oral hygiene (bacterial plaque and/or calculus)
- Patient may report an episode of trauma (especially for lesions on labial mucosa, tongue, and buccal mucosa)

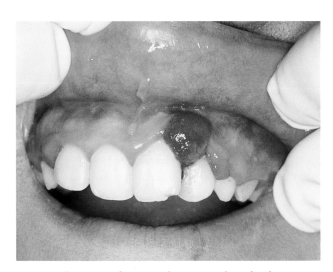

A pyogenic granuloma on the gingiva

DIAGNOSTIC STEPS

- Microscopic examination is necessary to confirm the diagnosis and rule out metastatic carcinoma

TREATMENT RECOMMENDATIONS

- Local surgical excision
- Treat local factors (remove bacterial plaque and/or calculus)

CLINICAL SIGNIFICANCE

- Lesions occasionally recur
- Metastatic carcinoma can mimic pyogenic granuloma

DIFFERENTIAL DIAGNOSIS
(Solitary Gingival Lesions)

- Peripheral giant cell granuloma
- Peripheral ossifying fibroma
- Metastatic carcinoma

PERIPHERAL GIANT CELL GRANULOMA

SYNONYMS

- Giant Cell Epulis

ETIOLOGY

- A reactive hyperplasia containing osteoclast-like multi-nucleated giant cells that develops in response to local irritating factors (bacterial plaque and/or calculus)

TYPICAL VISUAL CUES

- A solitary, circumscribed, red nodule with a broad (sessile) or narrow (pedunculated) base

- The surface is commonly ulcerated

- Occurs exclusively on gingiva

- Dental radiographs may show erosion of adjacent alveolar bone

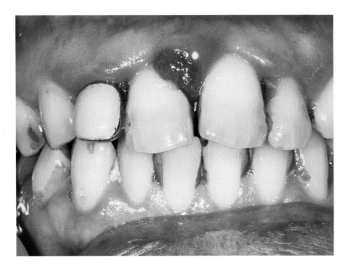

A peripheral giant cell granuloma on the gingiva

OTHER USEFUL CLINICAL INFORMATION

- Firm to palpation

- Usually painless

- Persistent (chronic)

- More common in women

- Often associated with poor oral hygiene (bacterial plaque and/or calculus)

DIFFERENTIAL DIAGNOSIS

- Pyogenic granuloma

- Peripheral ossifying fibroma

- Metastatic carcinoma

DIAGNOSTIC STEPS

- Microscopic examination necessary to confirm diagnosis and rule out metastatic carcinoma

TREATMENT RECOMMENDATIONS

- Local surgical excision

- Treat local factors (remove bacterial plaque and/or calculus)

CLINICAL SIGNIFICANCE

- Reported recurrence rate of approximately 10%

- Can occasionally mimic "brown tumor" of hyperparathyroidism

- Metastatic carcinoma can mimic peripheral giant cell granuloma

PERIPHERAL OSSIFYING FIBROMA

SYNONYMS

- Peripheral Fibroma with Calcifications

ETIOLOGY

- A reactive hyperplasia similar to a pyogenic granuloma with focal calcifications

TYPICAL VISUAL CUES

- A solitary, circumscribed, red to pink nodule with a broad (sessile) or narrow (pedunculated) base

- The surface can be smooth or ulcerated

- Occurs exclusively on gingiva (most often in the incisor-cuspid area)

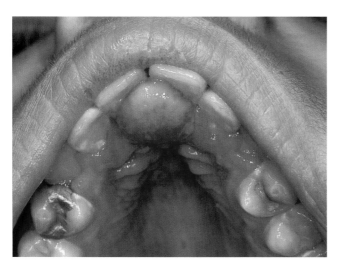

**A peripheral ossifying fibroma
on the marginal gingiva**

OTHER USEFUL CLINICAL INFORMATION

- Firm to palpation

- Usually painless

- Persistent (chronic)

- More common in women

- More common in adults

DIFFERENTIAL DIAGNOSIS

- Pyogenic granuloma

- Peripheral giant cell granuloma

- Fibroma

- Metastatic carcinoma

DIAGNOSTIC STEPS

- Microscopic examination necessary to confirm diagnosis and rule out metastatic carcinoma

TREATMENT RECOMMENDATIONS

- Local surgical excision

- Treat local factors (remove bacterial plaque and/or calculus)

CLINICAL SIGNIFICANCE

- Reported recurrence rate of approximately 15%

- Metastatic carcinoma can mimic peripheral ossifying fibroma

FIBROMA

SYNONYMS

- Irritation Fibroma
- Traumatic Fibroma

ETIOLOGY

- A reactive hyperplasia of fibrous connective tissue in response to trauma or local irritation (bacterial plaque and/or calculus)
- Gingival lesions may represent fibrosis of a pre-existing pyogenic granuloma

TYPICAL VISUAL CUES

- Solitary, circumscribed, pink nodule with a broad (sessile) base
- Covered with smooth mucosa unless secondarily traumatized (then calloused or ulcerated)
- Occurs most often on buccal mucosa, labial mucosa, tongue, and gingiva

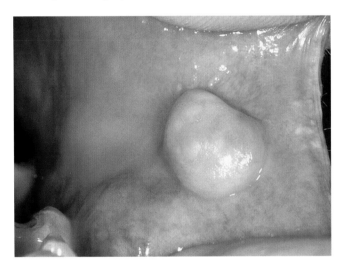

A fibroma on the buccal mucosa

DIFFERENTIAL DIAGNOSIS

- A lesion on buccal mucosa or tongue can mimic a benign neoplasm such as a neuroma or neurofibroma
- A lesion on labial mucosa can mimic a mucocele

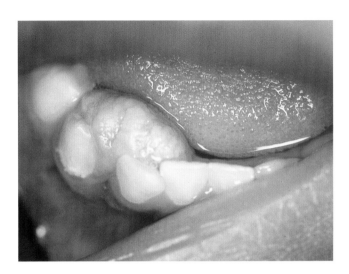

A fibroma on the gingiva

DIAGNOSTIC STEPS

- Microscopic examination necessary to confirm the diagnosis

TREATMENT RECOMMENDATIONS

- Local surgical excision

OTHER USEFUL CLINICAL INFORMATION

- Firm to palpation
- Usually painless
- Persistent (chronic)
- Patient may report a history of trauma (especially for buccal mucosa, labial mucosa, and tongue lesions)
- Gingival lesions may be associated with bacterial plaque and/or calculus
- Patient may report a pre-existing pyogenic granuloma

CLINICAL SIGNIFICANCE

- Recurrence unlikely if adequate excision
- Multiple oral mucosal fibromas can be a component of multiple hamartoma (Cowden's syndrome) and tuberous sclerosis
- Other components of Cowden's syndrome include skin tumors and breast cancer
- Other components of tuberous sclerosis include multiple skin tumors, seizures, and mental retardation

EPULIS FISSURATUM

SYNONYMS

- Denture Epulis

ETIOLOGY

- A reactive hyperplasia of fibrous connective tissue caused by chronic irritation from a denture flange

TYPICAL VISUAL CUES

- A circumscribed, pink nodule with a broad (sessile) base

- The nodule is often creased by a trough produced by the denture flange

- The surface is smooth unless secondarily traumatized (then calloused or ulcerated)

- Occurs most often on the labial surface of the maxillary alveolar ridge or the lingual surface of the mandibular alveolar ridge

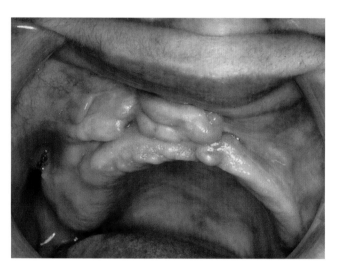

An epulis fissuratum on the labial surface of the maxillary alveolar ridge

OTHER USEFUL CLINICAL INFORMATION

- Firm to palpation

- Usually painless

- Persistent (chronic)

- The patient has usually worn the same dentures for many years (alveolar bone as resorption allows the denture flange to impinge on adjacent soft tissues)

DIFFERENTIAL DIAGNOSIS

- Because of its characteristic clinical presentation, epulis fissuratum is infrequently confused with other soft tissue swellings included in this section

- Ulcerated lesions can mimic squamous cell carcinoma

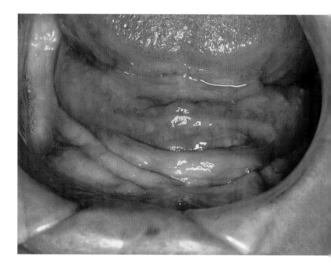

An epulis fissuratum on the lingual surface of the mandibular alveolar ridge

DIAGNOSTIC STEPS

- Microscopic examination is necessary to confirm the diagnosis and rule out squamous cell carcinoma

TREATMENT RECOMMENDATIONS

- Local surgical excision

- Reline existing denture or fabricate a new denture

CLINICAL SIGNIFICANCE

- Often associated with denture stomatitis and/or inflammatory papillary hyperplasia

- Persistent lesions thought to be denture-related should always be viewed with suspicion in the mouths of individuals at risk for oral cancer (those who use tobacco and alcohol)

MUCOCELE

SYNONYMS

- Mucous Escape Reaction

- Mucous Extravasation Phenomenon

ETIOLOGY

- Local trauma damages the excretory duct of a minor salivary gland

- Saliva escapes into the adjacent connective tissue causing a chronic inflammatory reaction

TYPICAL VISUAL CUES

- Solitary, circumscribed, nodule with a broad (sessile) base

- Superficial lesions are typically blue in color, while deeper lesions are pink

- The surface is usually smooth unless secondarily traumatized (then calloused or ulcerated)

- Occurs most often on the lower lip

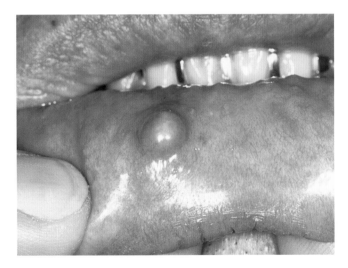

A mucocele on the mandibular labial mucosa

OTHER USEFUL CLINICAL INFORMATION

- Soft to palpation

- Usually painless

- Persistent (chronic)

- May occasionally fluctuate in size

- Patient often reports a history of trauma (usually biting injury)

DIFFERENTIAL DIAGNOSIS

- Fibroma

- Neuroma

- Neurofibroma

- Hemangioma

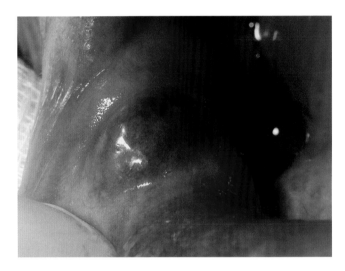

A mucocele on the mandibular labial mucosa

DIAGNOSTIC STEPS

- Microscopic examination necessary to confirm the diagnosis

TREATMENT RECOMMENDATIONS

- Local surgical excision

- Remove minor salivary glands at site to reduce likelihood of recurrence

CLINICAL SIGNIFICANCE

- Recurrence likely if minor salivary glands at the wound edges are not removed

RANULA

ETIOLOGY

- Usually caused by a sialolith (salivary duct stone) or local trauma to the duct of the submandibular salivary gland (Wharton's duct)

- Saliva escapes into the connective tissue of the floor of the mouth causing a chronic inflammatory reaction

TYPICAL VISUAL CUES

- Circumscribed, blue, sessile nodule usually covered with smooth mucosa

- Occurs in the floor of the mouth away from the midline

- May occasionally extend below the mylohyoid muscle to produce a swelling in the upper neck (plunging ranula)

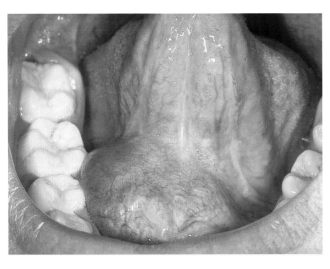

A ranula on the floor of the mouth

(From Newland JR, Fasser CE, and Smith QW, *Physician Assistant*, 1983, 7(1):88-99)

OTHER USEFUL CLINICAL INFORMATION

- Soft to palpation

- Usually painless

- Persistent (chronic)

- Patient may report a history of local trauma

DIFFERENTIAL DIAGNOSIS

- Hemangioma

- Lymphangioma

- Lymphoid hyperplasia

- Oral lymphoepithelial cyst

- Salivary gland neoplasms

DIAGNOSTIC STEPS

- Microscopic examination is necessary to confirm the diagnosis

TREATMENT RECOMMENDATIONS

- Marsupialization

- Removal of the submandibular glandular tissue may be necessary

PARULIS

SYNONYMS

- Gum Boil

ETIOLOGY

- A soft tissue (gingival) extension of an abscess originating from the apex of a tooth root (periapical abscess), or from periodontal tissues (periodontal abscess)

TYPICAL VISUAL CUES

- Circumscribed, erythematous, gingival mass

- Fistula with purulent discharge may be present

- Usually located on the buccal gingiva

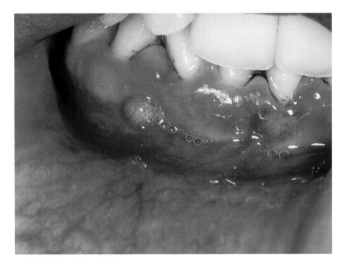

A parulis secondary to a periodontal abscess

OTHER USEFUL CLINICAL INFORMATION

- The patient may describe acute pain associated with a tooth (exacerbated by percussion) or from inflamed gingival tissue

- A periapical radiograph may show a circumscribed lesion at the root apex

- Periodontal probing may demonstrate the presence of a periodontal pocket

DIFFERENTIAL DIAGNOSIS

- Actinomycosis

- Pyogenic granuloma

- Gingival cyst of the adult

DIAGNOSTIC STEPS

- A periapical radiograph should be obtained to determine if a lesion is present at the apex of a tooth or if alveolar bone loss is present

- Electrical pulp testing should be performed to determine if the suspected tooth is nonvital

- Microscopic examination may be necessary to confirm the diagnosis

TREATMENT RECOMMENDATIONS

- Conventional endodontic therapy/apical surgery if indicated. Antibiotic therapy with Penicillin (*on page 145*), Amoxicillin (*on page 135*), Amoxicillin and Clavulanate Potassium (Augmentin® *on page 135*), or Metronidazole (Flagyl® *on page 144*) may be appropriate

- Periodontal therapy

ACTINOMYCOSIS

SYNONYMS

- Lumpy Jaw

ETIOLOGY

- A soft tissue swelling caused by an infection with the bacteria, *Actinomyces israelii*

- The most common form of infection is cervicofacial

- The initial site of infection is an area of soft tissue injury, a periodontal pocket, a periapical abscess, or an extraction site

TYPICAL VISUAL CUES

- Cutaneous swelling with fistula formation

- Yellow colonies of organisms called sulfur granules exude from the fistula

- Swelling occurs most often at the inferior border of the mandible

- Can also present as a gingival swelling

- Dental radiographs may show a periapical radiolucency (periapical abscess) associated with a nonvital tooth

DIFFERENTIAL DIAGNOSIS

- Because of its characteristic clinical presentation, actinomycosis is infrequently confused with other soft tissue swellings

- A gingival lesion can mimic a parulis

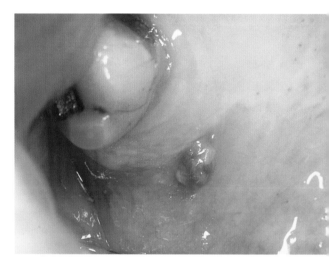

A gingival swelling secondary to actinomycosis

DIAGNOSTIC STEPS

- A bacterial culture (less than 50% are positive)

- Microscopic examination may be necessary to confirm diagnosis

TREATMENT RECOMMENDATIONS

- Treat infected tooth (conventional endodontics, apical surgery, or extraction)

- Appropriate antibiotic therapy, generally long-term (4-6 weeks), high-dose (10-20 million units/day) of intravenous penicillin

- May require drainage and debridement

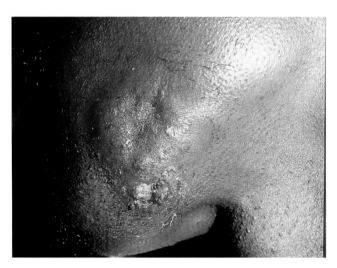

Cutaneous actinomycosis with sulfur granules

OTHER USEFUL CLINICAL INFORMATION

- Persistent

- Patient may describe pain of odontogenic or periodontal origin

LIPOMA

ETIOLOGY

- A benign neoplasm of fat

- May also represent a reaction of fat to local trauma

TYPICAL VISUAL CUES

- A solitary, circumscribed, nodule with a broad (sessile) base

- Usually covered with smooth mucosa

- Superficial lesions are typically yellow in color, while deeper lesions are pink

- Occurs most often on the buccal mucosa, ventral tongue, and floor of the mouth

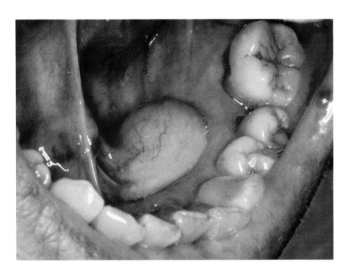

A lipoma on the floor of the mouth

OTHER USEFUL CLINICAL INFORMATION

- Soft to palpation

- Usually painless

- Persistent (chronic)

DIFFERENTIAL DIAGNOSIS

- Fibroma

- Neuroma

- Neurofibroma

- Lymphoid hyperplasia

- Oral lymphoepithelial cyst

- Salivary gland neoplasms

DIAGNOSTIC STEPS

- Microscopic examination necessary to confirm the diagnosis

TREATMENT RECOMMENDATIONS

- Local surgical excision

CLINICAL SIGNIFICANCE

- Recurrence unlikely

HEMANGIOMA

ETIOLOGY

- Benign neoplasm of the endothelial cells that form blood vessels

- Can be present at birth (congenital) or acquired later in life

TYPICAL VISUAL CUES

- Circumscribed, red to blue nodule with a broad (sessile) base

- Usually covered with smooth mucosa

- Solitary or multiple

- Digital pressure may cause the lesion to blanch

- Occur most often on the tongue, lips, and buccal mucosa

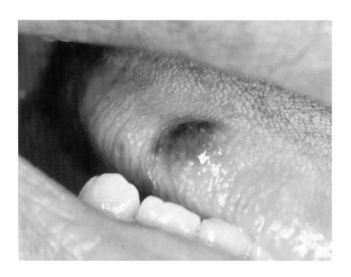

A hemangioma on the lateral tongue

OTHER USEFUL CLINICAL INFORMATION

- Soft to palpation

- Usually painless

- Congenital lesions may regress with time

- Acquired lesions tend to be persistent (chronic)

DIFFERENTIAL DIAGNOSIS

- Mucocele

- Hematoma

- Pyogenic granuloma

- Lymphangioma

DIAGNOSTIC STEPS

- Microscopic examination necessary to confirm the diagnosis

TREATMENT RECOMMENDATIONS

- Local surgical excision, laser therapy, and embolization

CLINICAL SIGNIFICANCE

- Multiple hemangiomas are a component of encephalo-trigeminal angiomatosis (Sturge-Weber syndrome)

- Other components of the syndrome include hemangiomas involving the skin of the face and the brain

LYMPHANGIOMA

ETIOLOGY

- A benign neoplasm of the endothelial cells that form lymphatic vessels

- Can be present at birth (congenital) or acquired later in life

TYPICAL VISUAL CUES

- Circumscribed, sessile, blue nodule with a broad (sessile) base

- Usually covered with smooth mucosa

- Occasionally, the lesions are more diffuse and exhibit a pebbly (multinodular) surface

- The tongue is the most common site of involvement

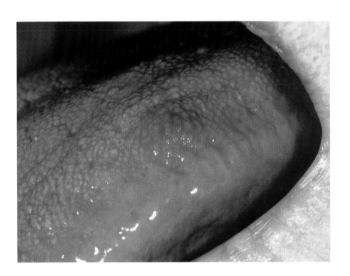

A lymphangioma on the lateral tongue

OTHER USEFUL CLINICAL INFORMATION

- Soft to palpation

- Usually painless

DIFFERENTIAL DIAGNOSIS

- Mucocele

- Hemangioma

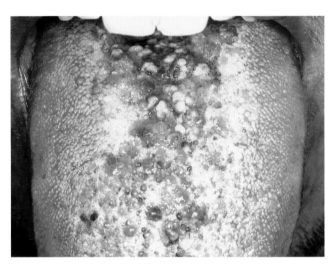

A lymphangioma on the dorsal tongue exhibiting a multinodular surface

DIAGNOSTIC STEPS

- Microscopic examination is necessary to confirm the diagnosis

TREATMENT RECOMMENDATIONS

- Local surgical excision

CLINICAL SIGNIFICANCE

- A common cause of enlarged tongue (macroglossia) in children

NEUROMA

SYNONYMS

- Traumatic Neuroma
- Amputation Neuroma

ETIOLOGY

- Caused by traumatic injury to a nerve bundle
- The nerve bundle proliferates to produce a mass in response to the trauma
- The precipitating injury is often secondary to tooth extraction

TYPICAL VISUAL CUES

- Solitary, circumscribed, pink nodule with a broad (sessile) base
- Usually covered with smooth mucosa
- Occurs most often in the mucosa over the mental foramen area (caused by injury to the mental nerve during extraction of teeth in the area)
- Occasionally involves the dorsal tongue

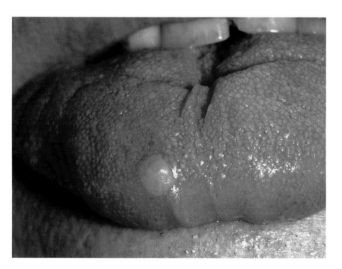

A traumatic neuroma on the tongue

OTHER USEFUL CLINICAL INFORMATION

- Lesions associated with the mental nerve are usually painful
- Pain can be referred along the inferior alveolar nerve
- Patient may report a history of trauma (such as tooth extraction)

DIFFERENTIAL DIAGNOSIS

- Fibroma
- Neurofibroma

DIAGNOSTIC STEPS

- Microscopic examination necessary to confirm the diagnosis

TREATMENT RECOMMENDATIONS

- Local surgical excision

CLINICAL SIGNIFICANCE

- Multiple oral mucosal neuromas are a component of multiple endocrine neoplasia syndrome (MEN)-type III
- Other components of MEN-type III are pheochromocytoma (a benign neoplasm of the adrenal gland) and medullary carcinoma of the thyroid gland

NEUROFIBROMA

ETIOLOGY

- A benign neoplasm of neurofibroblasts (the cells that form the supporting structure for nerves)

TYPICAL VISUAL CUES

- Solitary, circumscribed, pink nodule with a broad (sessile) base

- Usually covered with smooth mucosa

- Occurs most often on the tongue and buccal mucosa

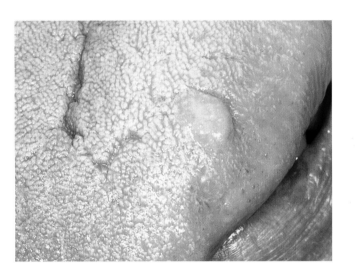

A neurofibroma on the dorsal tongue

OTHER USEFUL CLINICAL INFORMATION

- Firm to palpation
- Usually painless

DIFFERENTIAL DIAGNOSIS

- Fibroma

- Neuroma

DIAGNOSTIC STEPS

- Microscopic examination necessary to confirm the diagnosis

TREATMENT RECOMMENDATIONS

- Local surgical excision

CLINICAL SIGNIFICANCE

- Multiple oral mucosal neurofibromas are a component of neurofibromatosis (Von Recklinghausen's disease of skin)

- Other components of the syndrome include multiple cutaneous neurofibromas and pigmented skin lesions called cafe-au-lait macules

- As many as 15% of patients with the syndrome will develop neurofibrosarcomas

LYMPHOID HYPERPLASIA

SYNONYMS

- Hyperplastic Lymphoid Aggregates

ETIOLOGY

- Reactive hyperplasia of lymphoid aggregates in response to an antigenic challenge

TYPICAL VISUAL CUES

- Solitary or multiple, circumscribed, pink or yellow, sessile nodules covered with smooth mucosa

- Typically involves lymphoid aggregates located in the oropharynx, lateral tongue, floor of mouth, or soft palate

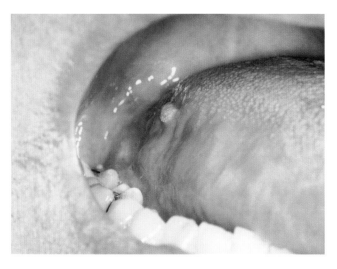

Lymphoid hyperplasia on the posterior lateral tongue

OTHER USEFUL CLINICAL INFORMATION

- Painless

- Persistent

- More common in adults

DIFFERENTIAL DIAGNOSIS

- Oral lymphoepithelial cyst

- Lipoma

- Ranula

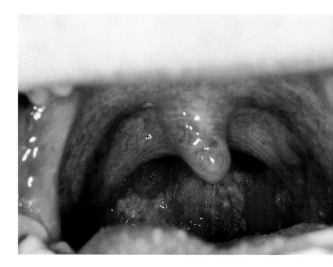

Lymphoid hyperplasia on the oropharynx

DIAGNOSTIC STEPS

- Microscopic examination necessary to confirm the diagnosis

TREATMENT RECOMMENDATIONS

- Once the diagnosis is confirmed, no other treatment necessary

CLINICAL SIGNIFICANCE

- Lymphoid hyperplasia is innocuous

ORAL LYMPHOEPITHELIAL CYST

ETIOLOGY

- A cyst that develops from epithelium entrapped in oral lymphoid tissue

TYPICAL VISUAL CUES

- A solitary, circumscribed, yellow-tan, sessile nodule covered with intact mucosa

- Most common sites include floor of the mouth, ventral tongue, and soft palate

DIFFERENTIAL DIAGNOSIS

- Lymphoid hyperplasia

- Lipoma

- Ranula

DIAGNOSTIC STEPS

- Microscopic examination necessary to confirm the diagnosis

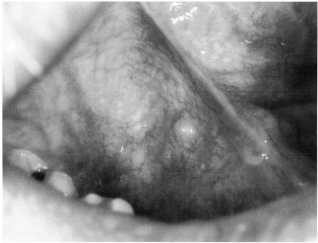

Oral lymphoepithelial cyst on the ventral tongue

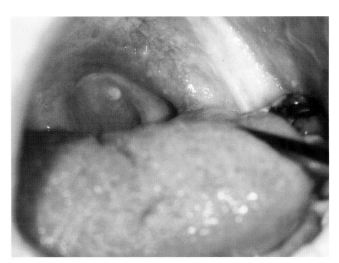

Oral lymphoepithelial cyst on the soft palate

OTHER USEFUL CLINICAL INFORMATION

- Painless

- Persistent

- More common in young adults

TREATMENT RECOMMENDATIONS

- Once the diagnosis is confirmed, no other treatment necessary

CLINICAL SIGNIFICANCE

- Oral lymphoepithelial cyst is innocuous

GINGIVAL CYST OF THE ADULT

ETIOLOGY

- A cyst that develops from epithelial rests of the dental lamina

TYPICAL VISUAL CUES

- A solitary, bluish, sessile mass covered with intact mucosa

- Occurs most often in the mandibular cuspid-premolar area

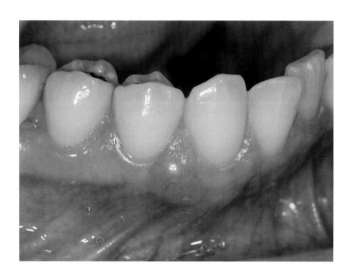

Gingival cyst of the adult

OTHER USEFUL CLINICAL INFORMATION

- Painless

- Persistent

- More common in adults

DIFFERENTIAL DIAGNOSIS

- Parulis

DIAGNOSTIC STEPS

- Microscopic examination necessary to confirm the diagnosis

TREATMENT RECOMMENDATIONS

- Local surgical excision

CLINICAL SIGNIFICANCE

- Gingival cyst of the adult is an innocuous lesion

CHEILITIS GLANDULARIS

ETIOLOGY

- Chronic inflammation of minor salivary glands in the lower lip

- Contributory factors include chronic sun exposure, tobacco exposure, infection, poor oral hygiene, and genetic predisposition

TYPICAL VISUAL CUES

- Diffuse enlargement of the lower lip

- Overlying mucosa often erythematous

- Inflamed openings of minor salivary gland ducts appear as red dots

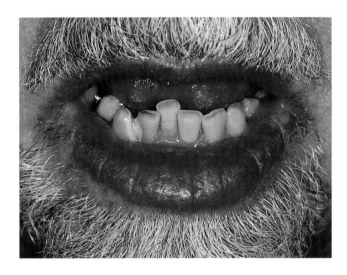

Cheilitis glandularis involving the lower lip

OTHER USEFUL CLINICAL INFORMATION

- May be painful

- More common in adult males

- Lower lip firm to palpation

DIFFERENTIAL DIAGNOSIS

- Because of its characteristic clinical appearance, cheilitis glandularis is infrequently confused with other soft tissue enlargements included in this section

DIAGNOSTIC STEPS

- Definitive diagnosis can usually be made on the basis of clinical presentation

- Biopsy may be necessary to rule out premalignant changes

TREATMENT RECOMMENDATIONS

- Topical applications of sunscreen

- Vermilionectomy in refractory cases

CLINICAL SIGNIFICANCE

- Cheilitis glandularis increases the risk of squamous cell carcinoma

BENIGN SALIVARY GLAND NEOPLASMS

ETIOLOGY

- A benign neoplasm of one or more components of salivary gland tissue

TYPICAL VISUAL CUES

- Solitary, circumscribed, pink mass with a broad (sessile) base

- Usually covered with smooth mucosa

- Occur most often on the hard palate away from the midline

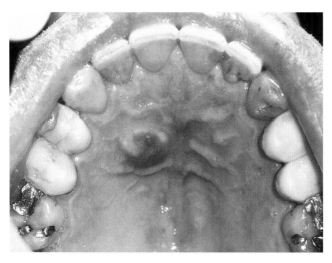

**A benign salivary gland neoplasm
on the hard palate**

OTHER USEFUL CLINICAL INFORMATION

- Usually painless

- Persistent (chronic)

DIFFERENTIAL DIAGNOSIS

- Benign connective tissue neoplasms

- Malignant salivary gland neoplasms

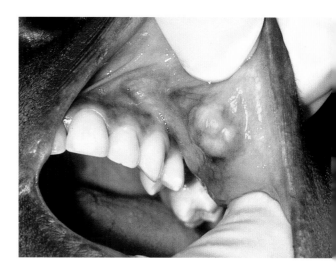

**A benign salivary gland neoplasm
on the buccal mucosa**

DIAGNOSTIC STEPS

- Microscopic examination is necessary to confirm the diagnosis

TREATMENT RECOMMENDATIONS

- Local surgical excision

CLINICAL SIGNIFICANCE

- Some benign salivary gland neoplasms have the potential to become malignant

DRUG-INDUCED GINGIVAL HYPERPLASIA

ETIOLOGY

- Gingival enlargement caused by a variety of drugs including phenytoin (Dilantin®), calcium channel blockers, and cyclosporine

- Exacerbated by local factors (bacterial plaque and calculus)

TYPICAL VISUAL CUES

- Generalized, pink, nodular enlargement of the attached gingiva

- Affects the anterior facial gingiva most often

- May completely obscure the teeth

- In the presence of significant local factors (bacterial plaque and calculus), the involved gingiva is red and bleeds easily

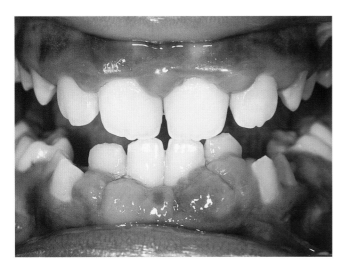

Drug-induced gingival hyperplasia in a patient using phenytoin

OTHER USEFUL CLINICAL INFORMATION

- Firm to palpation

- Usually painless

- Persistent (chronic)

- Phenytoin (Dilantin®) hyperplasia more common in children and young adults

- Hyperplasia secondary to calcium channel blockers and cyclosporine more common in adults

DIFFERENTIAL DIAGNOSIS

- Pregnancy gingivitis

- Leukemic gingivitis

DIAGNOSTIC STEPS

- The medical history will often reveal that the patient uses one of the offending drugs

- Microscopic examination will help to confirm the diagnosis

TREATMENT RECOMMENDATIONS

- Substitute another drug, if possible

- Remove local factors (bacterial plaque and calculus)

- Gingivectomy to remove excessive tissue

LEUKEMIC GINGIVAL INFILTRATE

SYNONYMS

- Leukemic Gingivitis

ETIOLOGY

- Gingival involvement caused by a proliferation of malignant white blood cells (monocytes, myelocytes, or lymphocytes)

- Occurs most often in acute monocytic leukemia

TYPICAL VISUAL CUES

- Spontaneous bleeding from the gingival sulcus

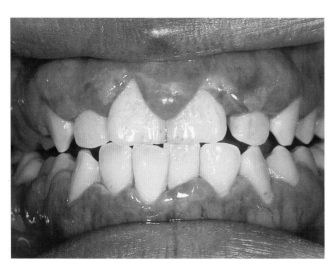

Diffuse gingival swelling in a patient with monocytic leukemia

OTHER USEFUL CLINICAL INFORMATION

- Usually firm to palpation

- Patient may also present with gingival ulcerations candidiasis, and recurrent intraoral herpes

- Dental radiographs may reveal alveolar bone loss and involved teeth may be mobile

- Patients may complain of fever, weight loss, and fatigue

DIFFERENTIAL DIAGNOSIS

- Pregnancy gingivitis

- Drug-induced gingival hyperplasia

DIAGNOSTIC STEPS

- Microscopic examination is necessary to confirm the diagnosis

TREATMENT RECOMMENDATIONS

- Treat leukemia with appropriate chemotherapy

CLINICAL SIGNIFICANCE

- Patient may develop oral mucositis

METASTATIC CARCINOMA

ETIOLOGY

- Caused by hematogenous (vascular) spread of a distant malignancy

- Most common primary sites are breast, lung, colon, and prostate

TYPICAL VISUAL CUES

- Solitary, circumscribed, red to pink nodule usually with a broad (sessile) base

- Surface is often ulcerated

- Occurs most frequently on gingiva

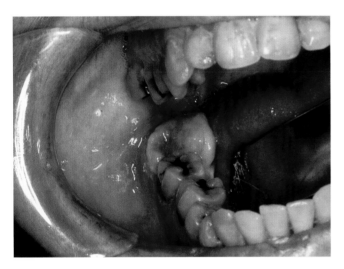

Metastatic colon cancer presenting as an ulcerated gingival swelling

OTHER USEFUL CLINICAL INFORMATION

- Firm to palpation

- Continuous enlargement

- Often associated with local discomfort

- More common in older adults

DIFFERENTIAL DIAGNOSIS

- Pyogenic granuloma

- Peripheral giant cell granuloma

- Peripheral ossifying fibroma

DIAGNOSTIC STEPS

- Microscopic examination necessary to confirm diagnosis

TREATMENT RECOMMENDATIONS

- Appropriate therapy for primary cancer

CLINICAL SIGNIFICANCE

- May be the first indication of disease

- Usually associated with a poor prognosis

ALPHABETICAL LISTING OF DRUGS
COMMONLY USED IN THE
TREATMENT OF ORAL SOFT TISSUE DISEASES

♦ Abreva® *see* Docosanol *on page 140*

Acetaminophen

Common US Brand Names Tylenol®
Therapeutic Category Analgesic, Non-narcotic; Antipyretic
Dosage Forms
Caplet
Capsule
Gelcap
Liquid
Suspension
Syrup
Tablet
Tablet, chewable
Strength
Caplet: 650 mg
Capsule: 500 mg
Gelcap: 650 mg
Liquid: 160 mg/5 mL
Suspension: 160 mg/5 mL
Syrup: 160 mg/5 mL
Tablet: 325 mg, 500 mg
Tablet, chewable: 80 mg
How Supplied Various commercial package sizes
Manufacturer Numerous
Use in Oral Medicine Treatment of postoperative pain
Mechanism of Action Inhibits the synthesis of prostaglandins in the CNS and peripherally blocks pain impulse generation; produces antipyresis by inhibition of hypothalamic heat-regulating center
Adult Dosing 325-650 mg (1-2 tablets) every 4-6 hours or 1000 mg 3-4 times/day
Maximum Adult Dose Do not exceed 4 g/day (4000 mg)
Pediatric Dosing Children <12 years: 10-15 mg/kg/dose every 4-6 hours as needed
Maximum Child Dose Do not exceed 5 doses (2.6 g) in 24 hours
Pregnancy Risk Factor B
Availability OTC
Comment Doses of acetaminophen >5 g/day for several weeks can produce severe, often fatal liver damage. Hepatotoxicity caused by acetaminophen is potentiated by chronic ethanol consumption. It has been reported that a combination of two quarts of whiskey a day with 8-10 acetaminophen tablets daily resulted in severe liver toxicity. People who consume ethanol at the same time that they use acetaminophen, even in therapeutic doses, are at risk of developing hepatotoxicity.

A study by Hylek, et al, suggested that the combination of acetaminophen with warfarin (Coumadin®) may cause enhanced anticoagulation. The following recommendations have been made by Hylek, et al, and supported by an editorial in *JAMA* by Bell.

Dose and duration of acetaminophen should be as low as possible, individualized and monitored

The study by Hylek reported the following:

For patients who reported taking the equivalent of at least 4 regular strength (325 mg) tablets for longer than a week, the odds of having an INR >6.0 were increased 10-fold above those not taking acetaminophen. Risk decreased with lower intakes of acetaminophen reaching a background level of risk at a dose of 6 or fewer 325 mg tablets per week.

Selected Readings
Bell WR, "Acetaminophen and Warfarin: Undesirable Synergy," *JAMA*, 1998, 279(9):702-3.
Dionne RA, Campbell RA, Cooper SA, et al, "Suppression of Postoperative Pain by Preoperative Administration of Ibuprofen in Comparison to Placebo, Acetaminophen, and Acetaminophen Plus Codeine," *J Clin Pharmacol*, 1983, 23(1):37-43.
Hylek EM, Heiman H, Skates SJ, et al, "Acetaminophen and Other Risk Factors for Excessive Warfarin Anticoagulation," *JAMA*, 1998, 279(9):657-62.
Lee WM, "Drug-Induced Hepatotoxicity," *N Engl J Med*, 1995, 333(17):1118-27.
Licht H, Seeff LB, and Zimmerman HJ, "Apparent Potentiation of Acetaminophen Hepatotoxicity by Alcohol," *Ann Intern Med*, 1980, 92(4):511.
McClain CJ, et al, "Potentiation of Acetaminophen Hepatotoxicity by Alcohol," *JAMA*, 1980, 244:251.
McClain CJ, Price S, Barve S, et al, "Acetaminophen Hepatotoxicity: An Update," *Curr Gastroenterol Rep*, 1999, 1(1):42-9.

Acyclovir Oral (Capsules or Tablets)

Common US Brand Names Zovirax®
Therapeutic Category Antiviral Agent, Oral
Dosage Forms
Capsule
Tablet
Strength
Capsule: 200 mg
Tablet: 400 mg, 800 mg

How Supplied Desired quantity from stock
Manufacturer Numerous
Use in Oral Medicine Treatment of initial and prophylaxis of recurrent mucosal and cutaneous herpes simplex (HSV-1 and HSV-2) infections

Note: The following bracketed information refers to uses that are not included in U.S. product labeling

Accepted
Herpes simplex (treatment): Topical acyclovir is indicated in the treatment of limited nonlife-threatening mucocutaneous herpes simplex virus (HSV-1 and HSV-2) infections in immunocompromised patients; however, systemic acyclovir is more effective and may be preferred

[Herpes zoster (treatment adjunct)]: Topical acyclovir is used as adjunctive therapy to improve cutaneous healing of localized herpes zoster in immunosuppressed persons being treated systemically with other treatment regimens for herpes zoster

Resistance to acyclovir, although currently of minor clinical significance, has been reported to develop with prolonged treatment in immunocompromised patients; resistance does not appear to be significant in patients with normal immune function

Unaccepted
Herpes genitalis (treatment): Although topical acyclovir is FDA-approved for the treatment of *initial* herpes genitalis infections caused by herpes simplex virus (HSV), the Centers for Disease Control (CDC) and USP medical experts do not recommend it for use, because oral acyclovir is considerably more effective

Topical acyclovir is not effective in the treatment of *recurrent* herpes genitalis or herpes febrilis (labialis) infections in nonimmunocompromised patients, although topical acyclovir may cause some reduction in the duration of viral shedding. Also, there is no evidence that topical acyclovir will prevent the transmission of herpes infection to others or that it will prevent recurrent infections in the absence of signs and symptoms of infection.
Mechanism of Action Inhibits DNA synthesis and viral replication by competing with deoxyguanosine triphosphate for viral DNA polymerase and incorporation into viral DNA
Adult Dosing Dosing weight should be based on the smaller of lean body weight or total body weight
Treatment of herpes simplex virus infections: A 200 mg every 4 hours while awake (5 times/day) for 10 days if initial episode; for 5 days if recurrence (begin at earliest signs of disease)
Treatment of varicella-zoster virus (chickenpox) infections: 600-800 mg/dose every 4 hours while awake (5 times/day) for 7-10 days or 1000 mg every 6 hours for 5 days
Treatment of herpes zoster (shingles) infections: Adults (immunocompromised): 800 mg every 4 hours (5 times/day) for 7-10 days
Chronic suppressive therapy for recurrent herpes simplex virus infections: 200 mg 3-4 times/day or 400 mg twice daily for up to 12 months, followed by re-evaluation
Pediatric Dosing Dosing weight should be based on the smaller of lean body weight or total body weight
Treatment of varicella-zoster virus (chickenpox) infections: 10-20 mg/kg/dose (up to 800 mg) 4 times/day for 5 days; begin treatment within the first 24 hours of rash onset
Treatment of herpes zoster (shingles) infections: Children (immunocompromised): 250-600 mg/m²/dose 4-5 times/day for 7-10 days
Pregnancy Risk Factor C
Availability Rx

Acyclovir Topical

Common US Brand Names Zovirax®
Therapeutic Category Antiviral Agent, Topical
Ingredients
Active: Acyclovir 5%; Other: Polyethylene glycol (PEG) base
Cream = aqueous cream base
Dosage Forms
Cream, topical
Ointment, topical
Strength 5%
How Supplied 3 g, 15 g tubes; cream: 2 g tubes
Manufacturer GSK Pharm
Use in Oral Medicine Treatment of initial and prophylaxis of recurrent mucosal and cutaneous herpes simplex (HSV-1 and HSV-2) infections

Note: The following bracketed information refers to uses that are not included in U.S. product labeling

Accepted
Herpes simplex (treatment): Topical acyclovir is indicated in the treatment of limited nonlife-threatening mucocutaneous herpes simplex virus (HSV-1 and HSV-2) infections in immunocompromised patients; however, systemic acyclovir is more effective and may be preferred

[Herpes zoster (treatment adjunct)]: Topical acyclovir is used as adjunctive therapy to improve cutaneous healing of localized herpes zoster in immunosuppressed persons being treated systemically with other treatment regimens for herpes zoster

Resistance to acyclovir, although currently of minor clinical significance, has been reported to develop with prolonged treatment in immunocompromised patients; resistance does not appear to be significant in patients with normal immune function

Unaccepted

Herpes genitalis (treatment): Although topical acyclovir is FDA-approved for the treatment of *initial* herpes genitalis infections caused by herpes simplex virus (HSV), the Centers for Disease Control (CDC) and USP medical experts do not recommend it for use, because oral acyclovir is considerably more effective

Topical acyclovir is not effective in the treatment of *recurrent* herpes genitalis or herpes febrilis (labialis) infections in nonimmunocompromised patients, although topical acyclovir may cause some reduction in the duration of viral shedding. Also, there is no evidence that topical acyclovir will prevent the transmission of herpes infection to others or that it will prevent recurrent infections in the absence of signs and symptoms of infection.

Mechanism of Action Inhibits DNA synthesis and viral replication by competing with deoxyguanosine triphosphate for viral DNA polymerase and incorporation into viral DNA

Adult Dosing Dosing weight should be based on the smaller of lean body weight or total body weight

Treatment of herpes simplex virus infections:

Ointment: $\frac{1}{2}$" ribbon of ointment for a 4" square surface area every 3 hours (6 times/day)

Cream: Apply 5 times/day for 4 days

Pregnancy Risk Factor C

Availability Rx

♦ Advil® *see* Ibuprofen OTC *on page 141*

♦ Aldara™ *see* Imiquimod *on page 141*

♦ Aleve® *see* Naproxen Sodium OTC *on page 144*

Amitriptyline

Therapeutic Category Antidepressant, Tricyclic (Tertiary Amine)
Dosage Forms Tablet
Strength 10 mg, 25 mg, 50 mg, 75 mg, 100 mg, 150 mg
How Supplied Desired quantity from stock
Manufacturer Various
Use in Oral Medicine Neuropathic pain
Mechanism of Action Increases the synaptic concentration of serotonin and/or norepinephrine in the central nervous system by inhibition of their reuptake by the presynaptic neuronal membrane
Adult Dosing 25-100 mg/day in evening and morning doses
Pregnancy Risk Factor C
Availability Rx

Amlexanox

Common US Brand Names Aphthasol™
Therapeutic Category Anti-inflammatory Agent, Locally-Applied
Ingredients Active: Amlexanox 50 mg/g; Other: Benzyl alcohol, gelatin, glyceryl monostearate, mineral oil, pectin, petrolatum, sodium carboxymethylcellulose
Dosage Forms Paste
Strength 5%
How Supplied 5 g tube
Manufacturer Block Drug
Use in Oral Medicine Treatment of aphthous ulcers (ie, canker sores); has been investigated in many allergic disorders
Mechanism of Action As a benzopyrano-bipyridine carboxylic acid derivative, amlexanox has anti-inflammatory and antiallergic properties; it inhibits chemical mediatory release of the slow-reacting substance of anaphylaxis (SRS-A) and may have antagonistic effects on interleukin-3
Adult Dosing Administer (0.5 cm – $\frac{1}{4}$") directly on ulcers 4 times/day following oral hygiene, after meals, and at bedtime
Pregnancy Risk Factor B
Availability Rx
Selected Readings

Binnie WH, Curro FA, Khandwala A, et al, "Amlexanox Oral Paste: A Novel Treatment That Accelerates the Healing of Aphthous Ulcers," *Compend Contin Educ Dent*, 1997, 18(11):1116-8, 1120-2, 1124.

Greer RO Jr, Lindenmuth JE, Juarez T, et al, "A Double-Blind Study of Topically Applied 5% Amlexanox in the Treatment of Aphthous Ulcers," *J Oral Maxillofac Surg*, 1993, 51(3):243-8.

Khandwala A, Van Inwegen RG, and Alfano MC, "5% Amlexanox Oral Paste, A New Treatment for Recurrent Minor Aphthous Ulcers: I. Clinical Demonstration of Acceleration of Healing and Resolution of Pain," *Oral Surg Oral Med Oral Pathol Oral Radiol Endod*, 1997, 83(2):222-30.

Khandwala A, Van Inwegen RG, Charney MR, et al, "5% Amlexanox Oral Paste, A New Treatment for Recurrent Minor Aphthous Ulcers: II. Pharmacokinetics and Demonstration of Clinical Safety," *Oral Surg Oral Med Oral Pathol Oral Radiol Endod*, 1997, 83(2):231-8.

Amoxicillin

Common US Brand Names Amoxil®; Trimox®
Therapeutic Category Antibiotic, Penicillin
Dosage Forms
Capsule
Powder for oral suspension
Tablet
Tablet, chewable
Strength
Capsule, as trihydrate: 250 mg, 500 mg
Powder for oral suspension, as trihydrate: 125 mg/5 mL, 250 mg/5 mL, 400 mg/5 mL
Tablet, chewable, as trihydrate: 125 mg, 250 mg, 400 mg
Tablet, film coated: 500 mg, 875 mg
How Supplied
Powder (when reconstituted): 80 mL, 100 mL, 150 mL
Tablets, capsules: Desired quantity from stock
Manufacturer Numerous
Use in Oral Medicine Antibiotic for standard prophylactic regimen for dental patients who are at risk
Mechanism of Action Interferes with bacterial cell wall synthesis during active multiplication, causing cell wall death and resultant bactericidal activity against susceptible bacteria
Adult Dosing
Subacute bacterial endocarditis prophylaxis (standard regimen): 2 g 1 hour before dental procedure with no follow-up dose
Joint replacement prophylaxis: 2 g 1 hour before dental procedure with no follow-up dose needed
Pediatric Dosing Subacute bacterial endocarditis prophylaxis (standard regimen): 50 mg/kg 1 hour before dental procedure with no follow-up dose needed
Maximum Child Dose Total children's dose should not exceed adult dose
Pregnancy Risk Factor B
Availability Rx
Selected Readings

Dajani AS, Taubert KA, Wilson W, et al, "Prevention of Bacterial Endocarditis. Recommendations by the American Heart Association," *JAMA* 1997, 277(22):1794-801.

Dajani AS, Taubert KA, Wilson W, et al, "Prevention of Bacterial Endocarditis: Recommendations by the American Heart Association," *J Am Dent Assoc* 1997, 128(8):1142-51.

Amoxicillin and Clavulanate Potassium

Common US Brand Names Augmentin®
Therapeutic Category Antibiotic, Penicillin
Dosage Forms
Powder for reconstitution as suspension
Tablet
Tablet, chewable
Tablet, extended release
Strength
Powder for reconstitution:
125 mg - 31.25 mg/5 mL
200 mg - 28.5 mg/5 mL
250 mg - 62.5 mg/5 mL
400 mg - 57 mg/5 mL
600 mg - 42.9 mg/5 mL
Tablet:
250 (250 mg - 125 mg)
500 (500 mg - 125 mg)
875 (875 mg - 125 mg)
Tablet, chewable:
125 (125 mg - 31.25 mg)
200 (200 mg - 28.5 mg)
250 (250 mg - 62.5 mg)
400 (400 mg - 57 mg)
Tablet, extended release:
Augmentin XR 1000 mg - 62.5 mg
How Supplied
Powder for suspension:
125: 75 mL, 100 mL, 150 mL
200: 50 mL, 75 mL, 100 mL
250: 75 mL, 100 mL, 150 mL
400: 50 mL, 75 mL, 100 mL
Tablet: Desired quantity from stock
(Continued)

Amoxicillin and Clavulanate Potassium *(Continued)*

Manufacturer SK Beecham Pharm

Use in Oral Medicine Treatment of orofacial infections when beta-lactamase-producing staphylococci and beta-lactamase-producing *Bacteroides* are present

Mechanism of Action Interferes with bacterial cell wall synthesis during active multiplication, causing cell wall death and resultant bactericidal activity against susceptible bacteria. Clavulanic acid binds and inhibits beta-lactamases that inactivate amoxicillin resulting in an antibiotic combination having an expanded spectrum of activity.

Adult Dosing Children >40 kg and Adults: 250-500 mg every 8 hours or 875 mg every 12 hours for at least 7 days

Maximum Adult Dose Maximum dose: 2 g/day

Pediatric Dosing <40 kg: 20-40 mg (amoxicillin)/kg/day in divided doses every 8 hours

Pregnancy Risk Factor B

Availability Rx

Comment In maxillary sinus, anterior nasal cavity, and deep neck infections, beta-lactamase-producing staphylococci and beta-lactamase-producing *Bacteroides* usually are present. In these situations, antibiotics that resist the beta-lactamase enzyme are indicated. Amoxicillin and clavulanic acid is administered orally for moderate infections. Ampicillin sodium and sulbactam sodium (Unasyn®) is administered parenterally for more severe infections.

♦ Amoxil® *see* Amoxicillin *on page 135*

Amphotericin B Cream 3%

Common US Brand Names Fungizone® Cream 3%

Therapeutic Category Antifungal Agent, Topical

Ingredients Unavailable

Dosage Forms Cream, topical

Strength 3%

How Supplied 20 g tube

Manufacturer Apothecon

Use in Oral Medicine Topically for cutaneous and mucocutaneous candidal infections

Mechanism of Action Binds to ergosterol altering cell membrane permeability in susceptible fungi and causing leakage of cell components with subsequent cell death

Adult Dosing Apply to affected areas 2-4 times/day for 1-4 weeks of therapy depending on nature and severity of infection

Pregnancy Risk Factor B

Availability Rx

♦ Anaprox® *see* Naproxen Sodium *on page 144*

♦ Anaprox DS® *see* Naproxen Sodium *on page 144*

♦ Anbesol® Maximum Strength [OTC] *see* Benzocaine Gel *on page 137*

Antiseptic Mouth Rinse

Common US Brand Names Listerine® Antiseptic

Therapeutic Category Antimicrobial Mouth Rinse; Antiplaque Agent; Mouthwash

Ingredients Active ingredients:

Listerine® Antiseptic: Thymol 0.064%, eucalyptus 0.092%, methyl salicylate 0.060%, menthol 0.042%, alcohol 26.9%, water, benzoic acid, poloxamer 407, sodium benzoate, caramel

Fresh Burst Listerine® Antiseptic: Thymol 0.064%, eucalyptus 0.092%, methyl salicylate 0.060%, menthol 0.042%, alcohol 26.9%, water, benzoic acid, poloxamer 407, sodium benzoate, flavoring, sodium, saccharin, sodium citrate, citric acid, D&C yellow #10, FD&C green #3

Cool Mint Listerine® Antiseptic: Thymol 0.064%, eucalyptus 0.092%, methyl salicylate 0.060%, menthol 0.042%, alcohol 26.9%, water, benzoic acid, poloxamer 407, sodium benzoate, flavoring, sodium, saccharin, sodium citrate, citric acid, FD&C green #3

Dosage Forms Liquid

Strength Commercial formula

How Supplied Various commercial sizes as Listerine® Antiseptic Cool Mint® Listerine® Antiseptic Fresh Burst®

Manufacturer Warner-Lambert Consumer

Use in Oral Medicine Reduces risk of secondary infection and may reduce duration of some oral ulcers; aids in the prevention and reduction of plaque and gingivitis; bad breath

Adult Dosing Rinse full strength for 30 seconds with 20 mL (²/₃ fluid oz or 4 teaspoonfuls) morning and night

Availability OTC

Comment The following information is endorsed on the label of the Listerine® products by the Council on Scientific Affairs, American Dental Association: "Listerine® Antiseptic has been shown to help prevent and reduce supragingival plaque accumulation and gingivitis when used in conscientiously applied program of oral hygiene and regular profession care. Its effect on periodontitis has not been determined."

♦ Aphthasol™ *see* Amlexanox *on page 135*

Aspirin

Therapeutic Category Salicylate

Dosage Forms
Caplet
Gelcap
Tablet
Tablet, chewable
Tablet, enteric coated

Strength
Caplet: 325 mg, 500 mg
Gelcap: 500 mg
Tablet: 325 mg
Tablet, chewable: 81 mg
Tablet, enteric coated: 81 mg, 325 mg, 500 mg, 650 mg

How Supplied Various commercial package sizes

Manufacturer Numerous

Use in Oral Medicine Treatment of postoperative pain

Mechanism of Action Inhibits prostaglandin synthesis by decreasing th activity of the enzyme, cyclo-oxygenase, which results in decreased forma tion of prostaglandin precursors, acts on the hypothalamic heat-regulatin center to reduce fever, blocks thromboxane synthetase action whic prevents formation of the platelet-aggregating substance thromboxane A

Adult Dosing Analgesic: 325-650 mg (1-2 tablets) every 4-6 hours

Maximum Adult Dose Up to 4 g/day

Pediatric Dosing Analgesic: 10-15 mg/kg/dose every 4-6 hours

Maximum Child Dose Up to a total of 60-80 mg/kg/24 hours

Pregnancy Risk Factor C (D if full-dose aspirin in 3rd trimester)

Availability OTC

Comment Patients taking one aspirin tablet daily as an antithrombotic an who require dental surgery should be given special consideration i consultation with the physician before removal of the aspirin relative t prevention of postoperative bleeding.

Attapulgite Suspension

Common US Brand Names Kaopectate®

Therapeutic Category Antidiarrheal

Dosage Forms Suspension

Strength 750 mg/15 mL

How Supplied 240 mL, 480 mL

Manufacturer Pharmacia/Upjohn

Use in Oral Medicine Sometimes used as a coating agent in combinatio with Benadryl® for treatment of oral ulcers

Adult Dosing Mix 50:50 with Benadryl® elixir for topical application

Pregnancy Risk Factor B

Availability OTC

♦ Augmentin® *see* Amoxicillin and Clavulanate Potassium *on page 135*

Azathioprine

Common US Brand Names Imuran®

Therapeutic Category Immunosuppressant Agent

Dosage Forms
Injection
Tablet

Strength
Injection, I.V.: 100 mg
Tablet: 50 mg

How Supplied
Injection, I.V.: 20 mL vial each containing 100 mg
Tablet: Desired quantity from stock

Manufacturer Glaxo Wellcome

Use in Oral Medicine Some practitioners advocate use in severe ulcera tive disorders; primarily used as an adjunct with other agents in preventio of rejection of solid organ transplants; also used in severe active rheuma toid arthritis unresponsive to other agents; azathioprine is an imidazoly derivative of 6-mercaptopurine

Mechanism of Action Antagonizes purine metabolism and may inhib synthesis of DNA, RNA, and proteins; may also interfere with cellula metabolism and inhibit mitosis

Adult Dosing I.V. dose is equivalent to oral dose
Renal transplantation: Oral, I.V.: 2-5 mg/kg/day to start, then 1-3 mg/k day maintenance
Rheumatoid arthritis: Oral: 1 mg/kg/day for 6-8 weeks; increase by 0.5 mg kg every 4 weeks until response or up to 2.5 mg/kg/day

Pediatric Dosing I.V. dose is equivalent to oral dose
Renal transplantation: Oral, I.V.: 2-5 mg/kg/day to start, then 1-3 mg/kg/day maintenance
Pregnancy Risk Factor D
Availability Rx

♦ Bacid® see Lactobacillus acidophilus and Lactobacillus bulgaricus on page 143

♦ Benadryl® see Diphenhydramine Liquid (Elixir and Syrup) on page 140

Benzocaine Gel

Common US Brand Names Anbesol® Maximum Strength [OTC]; Orabase®-B Maximum Strength
Therapeutic Category Local Anesthetic, Topical
Ingredients Active: Benzocaine 20%; Other: Ethanol, propylene glycol, ethylcellulose, flavor, sodium saccharin
Dosage Forms Gel
Strength 20% benzocaine
How Supplied 7 g tube
Manufacturer Colgate Oral, Lederle Consumer
Use in Oral Medicine Topical anesthesia to mucous membranes
Route of Administration Local application to mucous membranes
Mechanism of Action Ester local anesthetic blocks both the initiation and conduction of nerve impulses by decreasing the neuronal membrane's permeability to sodium ions, which results in inhibition of depolarization with resultant blockade of conduction
Adult Dosing
Mucous membranes: Dosage varies depending on area to be anesthetized and vascularity of tissues
Oral mouth/throat preparations: Do not administer for >2 days or in children <2 years of age, unless directed by a physician; refer to specific package labeling
Pediatric Dosing
Mucous membranes: Dosage varies depending on area to be anesthetized and vascularity of tissues
Oral mouth/throat preparations: Do not administer for >2 days or in children <2 years of age, unless directed by a physician; refer to specific package labeling
Pregnancy Risk Factor C
Availability OTC

Benzocaine Paste

Common US Brand Names Orabase®-B
Therapeutic Category Local Anesthetic, Topical
Ingredients Unavailable
Dosage Forms Paste
Strength 20%
How Supplied 5 g tube; 7 g tube; 15 g tube
Manufacturer Colgate Oral
Use in Oral Medicine Ester-type topical local anesthetic for temporary relief of pain associated with toothache, minor sore throat pain and canker sores
Mechanism of Action Local anesthetics bind selectively to the intracellular surface of sodium channels to block influx of sodium into the axon. As a result, depolarization necessary for action potential propagation and subsequent nerve function is prevented. The block at the sodium channel is reversible. When drug diffuses away from the axon, sodium channel function is restored and nerve propagation returns.
Adult Dosing
Mucous membranes: Dosage varies depending on area to be anesthetized and vascularity of tissues
Oral mouth/throat preparations: Do not administer for >2 days or in children <2 years of age, unless directed by a physician; refer to specific package labeling
Pediatric Dosing
Mucous membranes: Dosage varies depending on area to be anesthetized and vascularity of tissues
Oral mouth/throat preparations: Do not administer for >2 days or in children <2 years of age, unless directed by a physician; refer to specific package labeling
Pregnancy Risk Factor C
Availability OTC

♦ Biaxin® see Clarithromycin on page 138

Cephalexin

Common US Brand Names Keflex®
Therapeutic Category Antibiotic, Cephalosporin (First Generation)
Dosage Forms
Capsule
Powder for reconstitution as suspension
Tablet for oral suspension
Strength
Capsule: 250 mg, 500 mg
Powder for reconstitution: 125 mg/5 mL, 250 mg/5 mL
Tablet for oral suspension: 125 mg, 250 mg
How Supplied
Capsule / Tablet: Desired quantity from stock
Powder for suspension:
125 mg/5 mL: 100 mL, 200 mL
250 mg/5 mL: 100 mL, 200 mL
Manufacturer Numerous
Use in Oral Medicine An alternate antibiotic in treatment of orofacial infections in patients allergic to penicillins; susceptible bacteria including aerobic gram-positive bacteria and anaerobes. Also, an alternate antibiotic for prevention of bacterial endocarditis; individuals allergic to amoxicillin (penicillins) may receive cephalexin provided they have not had an immediate, local, or systemic IgE-mediated anaphylactic allergic reaction to penicillin. Also, antibiotic for premedication in patients not allergic to penicillin who may be at potential increased risk of hematogenous total joint infection.
Mechanism of Action Inhibits bacterial cell wall synthesis by binding to one or more of the penicillin-binding proteins (PBPs) which in turn inhibits the final transpeptidation step of peptidoglycan synthesis in bacterial cell walls, thus inhibiting cell wall biosynthesis. Bacteria eventually lyse due to ongoing activity of cell wall autolytic enzymes (autolysins and murein hydrolases) while cell wall assembly is arrested.
Adult Dosing 250-1000 mg every 6 hours
SBE prophylaxis: 2 g 1 hour before procedure with no follow-up dose needed
Joint prosthesis prophylaxis: 2 g 1 hour before procedure with no follow-up dose
Maximum Adult Dose 4 g/day
Pediatric Dosing 25-50 mg/kg/day every 6 hours; severe infections: 50-100 mg/kg/day in divided doses every 6 hours
SBE prophylaxis: 50 mg/kg orally 1 hour before procedure with no follow-up dose needed
Maximum Child Dose
Severe infections: Maximum: 3 g/24 hours
SBE prophylaxis: Total children's dose not to exceed adult dose
Pregnancy Risk Factor B
Availability Rx
Comment Cephalexin is effective against anaerobic bacteria, but the sensitivity of alpha-hemolytic Streptococcus vary; approximately 10% of strains are resistant. Nearly 70% are intermediately sensitive. Patients allergic to penicillins can use a cephalosporin; the incidence of cross-reactivity between penicillins and cephalosporins is 1% when the allergic reaction to penicillin is delayed. If the patient has a history of immediate reaction to penicillin, the incidence of cross-reactivity is 20%; cephalosporins are contraindicated in these patients.
Selected Readings
"Advisory Statement. Antibiotic Prophylaxis for Dental Patients With Total Joint Replacements. American Dental Association; American Academy of Orthopedic Surgeons," J Am Dent Assoc, 1997, 128(7):1004-8.
Dajani AS, Taubert KA, Wilson W, et al, "Prevention of Bacterial Endocarditis. Recommendations by the American Heart Association," JAMA 1997, 277(22):1794-801.
Dajani AS, Taubert KA, Wilson W, et al, "Prevention of Bacterial Endocarditis: Recommendations by the American Heart Association," J Am Dent Assoc 1997, 128(8):1142-51.

Cevimeline

Common US Brand Names Evoxac™
Therapeutic Category Cholinergic Agent
Dosage Forms Capsule
Strength 30 mg
How Supplied Desired quantity from stock
Manufacturer Snowbrand
Use in Oral Medicine Treatment of symptoms of dry mouth in patients with Sjögren's syndrome
Mechanism of Action Binds to muscarinic (cholinergic) receptors, causing an increase in secretion of exocrine glands (including salivary glands)
Adult Dosing 30 mg 3 times/day
Pregnancy Risk Factor C; there are no adequate or well-controlled studies in pregnant women. Use only if potential benefit justifies potential risk to the fetus; excretion in breast milk is unknown/not recommended.
Availability Rx
Comment May be taken with or without food; take with food if medicine causes upset stomach. May cause decreased visual acuity (particularly at night and in patients with central lens changes) and impaired depth perception; patients should be cautioned about driving at night or performing hazardous activities in reduced lighting.

Chlorhexidine Gluconate

Common US Brand Names Peridex®; PerioGard®
Therapeutic Category Antimicrobial Mouth Rinse; Antiplaque Agent
Dosage Forms Solution
Strength 0.12%
How Supplied 480 mL
Manufacturer Numerous
Use in Oral Medicine Antimicrobial dental rinse; chlorhexidine is active against gram-positive and gram-negative organisms, facultative anaerobes, aerobes, and yeast
Mechanism of Action The bactericidal effect of chlorhexidine is a result of the binding of this cationic molecule to negatively charged bacterial cell walls and extramicrobial complexes. At low concentrations, this causes an alteration of bacterial cell osmotic equilibrium and leakage of potassium and phosphorous resulting in a bacteriostatic effect. At high concentrations of chlorhexidine, the cytoplasmic contents of the bacterial cell precipitate and result in cell death.
Adult Dosing Oral rinse:
Precede use of solution by flossing and brushing teeth; completely rinse toothpaste from mouth. Swish 15 mL undiluted oral rinse around in mouth for 30 seconds, then expectorate. Caution patient not to swallow the medicine. Avoid eating for 2-3 hours after treatment. (The cap on bottle of oral rinse is a measure for 15 mL.)
When used as a treatment of gingivitis, the regimen begins with oral prophylaxis. Patient treats mouth with 15 mL chlorhexidine, swishes for 30 seconds, then expectorates. This is repeated twice daily (morning and evening). Patient should have a re-evaluation followed by a dental prophylaxis every 6 months.
Pregnancy Risk Factor B
Availability Rx

Clarithromycin

Common US Brand Names Biaxin®
Therapeutic Category Antibiotic, Macrolide
Dosage Forms
Granules for oral suspension
Tablet
Tablet, extended release
Strength
Granules for oral suspension: 125 mg/5 mL, 250 mg/5 mL
Tablet: 250 mg, 500 mg
Tablet, extended release: 500 mg
How Supplied Desired quantity from stock
Manufacturer Abbott Pharm
Use in Oral Medicine Alternate antibiotic in the treatment of common orofacial infections caused by aerobic gram-positive cocci and susceptible anaerobes; alternate antibiotic for the prevention of bacterial endocarditis in patients undergoing dental procedures
Mechanism of Action Exerts its antibacterial action by binding to 50S ribosomal subunit resulting in inhibition of protein synthesis. The 14-OH metabolite of clarithromycin is twice as active as the parent compound.
Adult Dosing 250-500 mg every 12 hours for 7 days; prevention of bacterial endocarditis: 500 mg 1 hour before procedure
Pediatric Dosing Prevention of bacterial endocarditis: 15 mg/kg orally 1 hour before procedure
Maximum Child Dose Total children's dose should not exceed adult dose
Pregnancy Risk Factor C
Availability Rx

♦ Cleocin® see Clindamycin on page 138

Clindamycin

Common US Brand Names Cleocin®
Therapeutic Category Acne Products; Antibiotic, Anaerobic; Antibiotic, Miscellaneous
Dosage Forms
Capsule, as hydrochloride
Granules, for oral solution as palmitate
Strength
Capsule: 150 mg, 300 mg
Granules for reconstitution: 75 mg/5 mL
How Supplied
Capsule: Desired quantity from stock
Granules, for reconstitution 100 mL:
125 mg/5 mL: 100 mL, 200 mL
250 mg/5 mL: 100 mL, 200 mL
Manufacturer Numerous
Use in Oral Medicine Alternate antibiotic, when amoxicillin cannot be used, for the standard regimen for prevention of bacterial endocarditis in patients undergoing dental procedures; an alternative to penicillin VK and erythromycin for treating orofacial infections; alternate antibiotic for prophylaxis for dental patients with total joint replacement
Mechanism of Action Reversibly binds to 50S ribosomal subunit preventing peptide bond formation thus inhibiting bacterial protein synthesis; bacteriostatic or bactericidal depending on drug concentration, infection site, and organism
Adult Dosing
Prevention of bacterial endocarditis in patients unable to take amoxicillin: 600 mg 1 hour before procedure with no follow-up dose needed
Orofacial infections: 150-450 mg every 6 hours for at least 7 days
Patients with prosthesis allergic to penicillin: 600 mg 1 hour before procedure with no follow-up dose
Maximum Adult Dose Orofacial infections: Maximum dose: 1.8 g/day
Pediatric Dosing
Prevention of bacterial endocarditis: 20 mg/kg orally 1 hour before procedure with no follow-up dose needed
Orofacial infections: 8-25 mg/kg in 3-4 equally divided doses
Pregnancy Risk Factor B
Availability Rx
Comment Clindamycin has not been shown to interfere with oral contraceptive activity; however, it reduces GI microflora, thus, oral contraceptive users should be advised to use additional methods of birth control. About 1% of clindamycin users develop pseudomembranous colitis. Symptoms may occur 2-9 days after initiation of therapy; however, it has never occurred with the 1-dose regimen of clindamycin used to prevent bacterial endocarditis.
Selected Readings
"Advisory Statement. Antibiotic Prophylaxis for Dental Patients With Total Joint Replacements. American Dental Association; American Academy of Orthopedic Surgeons," *J Am Dent Assoc*, 1997, 128(7):1004-8.
Dajani AS, Taubert KA, Wilson W, et al, "Prevention of Bacterial Endocarditis. Recommendations by the American Heart Association," *JAMA* 1997, 277(22):1794-801.
Dajani AS, Taubert KA, Wilson W, et al, "Prevention of Bacterial Endocarditis: Recommendations by the American Heart Association," *J Am Dent Assoc* 1997, 128(8):1142-51.

Clobetasol Propionate Ointment 0.05%

Common US Brand Names Temovate®
Therapeutic Category Corticosteroid, Topical (Very High Potency)
Ingredients Active: Clobetasol propionate 0.5 mg/g in a base of propylene glycol, sorbitan sesquiolate, and white petrolatum
Dosage Forms Ointment, topical
Strength 0.05%
How Supplied 15 g, 30 g, 45 g, 60 g tubes
Manufacturer Glaxo Derm
Use in Oral Medicine Short-term relief of inflammation of moderate to severe corticosteroid-responsive dermatosis (very high potency topical corticosteroid)
Mechanism of Action Stimulates the synthesis of enzymes needed to decrease inflammation, suppress mitotic activity, and cause vasoconstriction
Adult Dosing Apply twice daily for up to 2 weeks with no more than 50 g/week. Therapy should be discontinued when control is achieved; if no improvement is seen, reassessment of diagnosis may be necessary.
Maximum Adult Dose 50 g/week
Pregnancy Risk Factor C
Availability Rx

Clonazepam

Common US Brand Names Klonopin®
Therapeutic Category Benzodiazepine
Dosage Forms Tablet
Strength 0.5 mg, 1 mg, 2 mg
How Supplied Desired quantity from stock
Manufacturer Various
Use in Oral Medicine Burning mouth syndrome
Mechanism of Action The exact mechanism is unknown, but believed to be related to its ability to enhance the activity of GABA; suppresses the spike-and-wave discharge in absence seizures by depressing nerve transmission in the motor cortex
Adult Dosing 0.25-3 mg/day in evening and morning doses
Pregnancy Risk Factor D
Availability Rx

Clotrimazole Oral Troche

Common US Brand Names Mycelex®
Therapeutic Category Antifungal Agent, Oral Nonabsorbed
Ingredients Active: Clotrimazole 10 mg; Other: Dextrose, microcrystalline cellulose, povidone, magnesium stearate
Dosage Forms Troche, oral
Strength 10 mg

How Supplied 70s ea
Manufacturer Alza
Use in Oral Medicine Treatment of susceptible fungal infections, including oropharyngeal candidiasis; limited data suggests that the use of clotrimazole troches may be effective for prophylaxis against oropharyngeal candidiasis in neutropenic patients
Mechanism of Action Binds to phospholipids in the fungal cell membrane altering cell wall permeability resulting in loss of essential intracellular elements
Adult Dosing 10 mg troche dissolved slowly 5 times/day for 14 consecutive days
Pediatric Dosing >3 years: 10 mg troche dissolved slowly 5 times/day for 14 consecutive days
Pregnancy Risk Factor C
Availability Rx

Cyclophosphamide

Common US Brand Names Cytoxan®
Therapeutic Category Antineoplastic Agent, Alkylating Agent
Dosage Forms
  Powder for reconstitution
  Tablet
Strength
  Injection, powder for reconstitution:
    Cytoxan®: 500 mg, 1 g, 2 g [contains mannitol 75 mg per cyclophosphamide 100 mg]
  Tablet (Cytoxan®): 25 mg, 50 mg
How Supplied Desired quantity from stock
Manufacturer Various
Use in Oral Medicine Wegener's granulomatosis, systemic lupus erythematosus
Mechanism of Action Cyclophosphamide is an alkylating agent that prevents cell division by cross-linking DNA strands and decreasing DNA synthesis. It is a cell cycle phase nonspecific agent. Cyclophosphamide also possesses potent immunosuppressive activity. Cyclophosphamide is a prodrug that must be metabolized to active metabolites in the liver.
Adult Dosing Refer to individual protocols. Patients who are heavily pretreated with cytotoxic radiation or chemotherapy, or who have compromised bone marrow function may require a 33% to 50% reduction in initial dose.
  Usual dose:
    Oral: 50-100 mg/m^2/day as continuous therapy or 400-1000 mg/m^2 in divided doses over 4-5 days as intermittent therapy
    I.V.:
      Single doses: 400-1800 mg/m^2 (30-50 mg/kg) per treatment course (1-5 days) which can be repeated at 2- to 4-week intervals
      Continuous daily doses: 60-120 mg/m^2 (1-2.5 mg/kg) per day
Pregnancy Risk Factor D
Availability Rx

Cyclosporine

Common US Brand Names Gengraf®; Neoral®; Restasis™; Sandimmune®
Therapeutic Category Immunosuppressant Agent
Dosage Forms
  Capsule
  Emulsion, ophthalmic
  Solution for injection
  Solution, oral
Strength
  Capsule, soft gel, modified: 25 mg, 100 mg [contains castor oil, ethanol]
    Gengraf®: 25 mg, 100 mg [contains ethanol, castor oil, propylene glycol]
    Neoral®: 25 mg, 100 mg [contains dehydrated ethanol, corn oil, castor oil, propylene glycol]
  Capsule, soft gel, non-modified (Sandimmune®): 25 mg, 100 mg [contains dehydrated ethanol, corn oil]
  Emulsion, ophthalmic [preservative free, single-use vial] (Restasis™): 0.05% (0.4 mL) [contains glycerin, castor oil, polysorbate 80, carbomer 1342; 32 vials/box]
  Injection, solution, non-modified (Sandimmune®): 50 mg/mL (5 mL) [contains Cremophor® EL (polyoxyethylated castor oil), ethanol]
  Solution, oral, modified:
    Gengraf®: 100 mg/mL (50 mL) [contains castor oil, propylene glycol]
    Neoral®: 100 mg/mL (50 mL) [contains dehydrated ethanol, corn oil, castor oil, propylene glycol]
  Solution, oral, non-modified (Sandimmune®): 100 mg/mL (50 mL) [contains olive oil, ethanol]
How Supplied Desired quantity from stock
Manufacturer Various
Mechanism of Action Inhibition of production and release of interleukin II and inhibits interleukin II-induced activation of resting T-lymphocytes

Adult Dosing Note: Neoral® and Sandimmune® are not bioequivalent and cannot be used interchangeably
  Autoimmune diseases: 1-3 mg/kg/day
Pregnancy Risk Factor C
Availability Rx

♦ **Cytoxan**® *see* Cyclophosphamide *on page 139*

Dapsone

Therapeutic Category Antibiotic, Miscellaneous
Dosage Forms Tablet
Strength 25 mg, 100 mg
How Supplied Desired quantity from stock
Manufacturer Various
Use in Oral Medicine Used in lupus and in selected ulcerative conditions in consult with patient's physician
Mechanism of Action Competitive antagonist of para-aminobenzoic acid (PABA) and prevents normal bacterial utilization of PABA for the synthesis of folic acid
Adult Dosing Dermatitis herpetiformis: Oral: Initial: 50 mg/day, increase to 300 mg/day or higher to achieve full control. Reduce dosage to minimum level as soon as possible.
Pregnancy Risk Factor C
Availability Rx

♦ **Decadron**® **Elixir** *see* Dexamethasone Elixir 0.5 mL/5 mL *on page 139*

♦ **Deltasone**® *see* Prednisone *on page 145*

♦ **Denavir**™ **Cream** *see* Penciclovir Cream *on page 145*

Dexamethasone Elixir 0.5 mL/5 mL

Common US Brand Names Decadron® Elixir
Therapeutic Category Antiemetic; Anti-inflammatory Agent; Corticosteroid, Systemic
Dosage Forms Elixir
Strength 0.5 mg/5 mL
How Supplied 240 mL
Manufacturer Numerous
Use in Oral Medicine Treatment of a variety of oral diseases of allergic, inflammatory, or autoimmune origin
Mechanism of Action Decreases inflammation by suppression of migration of polymorphonuclear leukocytes and reversal of increased capillary permeability; suppresses normal immune response
Adult Dosing Anti-inflammatory: Swish 1 teaspoonful for 2 minutes 4 times/day. Instruct patient to expectorate excess to avoid systemic effect. Therapy should be discontinued when control is achieved. If no improvement is seen, reassessment of diagnosis may be necessary.
Pediatric Dosing Anti-inflammatory immunosuppressant: 0.08-0.3 mg/kg/day or 2.5-10 mg/m^2/day in divided doses every 6-12 hours; therapy should be discontinued when control is achieved; if no improvement is seen, reassessment of diagnosis may be necessary.
Pregnancy Risk Factor C
Availability Rx

♦ **Diflucan**® *see* Fluconazole Tablets *on page 140*

Diflunisal

Common US Brand Names Dolobid®
Therapeutic Category Analgesic, Non-narcotic; Nonsteroidal Anti-inflammatory Drug (NSAID), Oral
Dosage Forms Tablet
Strength 250 mg, 500 mg
How Supplied Desired quantity from stock
Manufacturer Merck
Use in Oral Medicine Treatment of postoperative pain
Mechanism of Action Inhibits prostaglandin synthesis by decreasing the activity of the enzyme, cyclo-oxygenase, which results in decreased formation of prostaglandin precursors
Adult Dosing 500-1000 mg followed by 250-500 mg every 8-12 hours
Maximum Adult Dose 1.5 g/day
Pregnancy Risk Factor C (D in third trimester)
Availability Rx
Comment The advantage of diflunisal as a pain reliever is its 12-hour duration of effect. In many cases, this long effect will ensure a full night sleep during the postoperative pain period.

DIPHENHYDRAMINE LIQUID (ELIXIR AND SYRUP)

Diphenhydramine Liquid (Elixir and Syrup)

Common US Brand Names Benadryl®
Therapeutic Category Antidote, Hypersensitivity Reactions; Antihistamine; Sedative
Dosage Forms Elixir, liquid as hydrochloride
Strength Elixir: 12.5 mg/5 mL; Liquid: 12.5 mg/5 mL
How Supplied 120 mL, 240 mL
Manufacturer Numerous
Use in Oral Medicine Symptomatic relief of allergic symptoms caused by histamine release which include nasal allergies and allergic dermatosis; also to produce local anesthesia through infiltration of mucous membranes
Mechanism of Action Competes with histamine for H_1-receptor sites on effector cells in the gastrointestinal tract, blood vessels, and respiratory tract
Adult Dosing 25-50 mg every 6-8 hours
Pediatric Dosing >10 kg: 12.5-25 mg 3-4 times/day
Maximum Child Dose 300 mg/day
Pregnancy Risk Factor C
Availability OTC
Comment 25-50 mg of diphenhydramine orally every 4-6 hours can be used to treat mild dermatologic manifestations of allergic reactions to penicillin and other antibiotics. Diphenhydramine is not recommended as local anesthetic for either infiltration route or nerve block since the vehicle has caused local necrosis upon injection. A 50:50 mixture of diphenhydramine liquid (12.5 mg/5 mL) in Kaopectate® or Maalox® is used as a local application for recurrent aphthous ulcers; swish 1 tablespoonful for 2 minutes 4 times/day.

Docosanol

Common US Brand Names Abreva®
Therapeutic Category Antiviral Agent, Topical
Ingredients Unavailable
Dosage Forms Cream
Strength 10%
How Supplied 0.07 oz
Manufacturer GSK Consumer
Use in Oral Medicine Treatment of herpes simplex of the face or lips
Mechanism of Action Prevents viral entry and replication at the cellular level
Adult Dosing Herpes simplex (face/lips): Topical: Apply 5 times/day to affected area of face or lips. Start at first sign of cold sore or fever blister and continue until healed.
Pediatric Dosing Herpes simplex: Children ≥12 years: Apply 5 times/day to affected area of face or lips. Start at first sign of cold sore or fever blister and continue until healed.
Availability OTC

♦ Dolobid® see Diflunisal on page 139

Doxepin

Common US Brand Names Sinequan®; Zonalon®
Therapeutic Category Antidepressant, Tricyclic (Tertiary Amine); Topical Skin Product
Dosage Forms
Capsule
Cream
Solution
Strength
Capsules: 10 mg, 25 mg, 50 mg, 75 mg, 100 mg
Cream: 5%, 30 g, 5 g
How Supplied Desired quantity from stock
Manufacturer Various
Use in Oral Medicine Burning mouth syndrome and neuropathic pain in cream form
Mechanism of Action Increases the synaptic concentration of serotonin and norepinephrine in the central nervous system by inhibition of their reuptake by the presynaptic neuronal membrane
Adult Dosing Apply locally 3-4 times/day
Pregnancy Risk Factor C
Availability Rx

Doxycycline Calcium Syrup

Common US Brand Names Vibramycin® Syrup
Therapeutic Category Antibiotic, Tetracycline Derivative
Dosage Forms Syrup, oral
Strength 50 mg/5 mL
How Supplied Desired quantity from stock
Manufacturer Pfizer

Use in Oral Medicine Treatment of periodontitis associated with presenc of *Actinobacillus actinomycetemcomitans* (AA); principally in the treatmer of infections caused by susceptible *Rickettsia*, *Chlamydia*, and *Myco plasma* along with uncommon susceptible gram-negative an gram-positive organisms. Reduces risk of secondary infections in som oral ulcers.
Mechanism of Action Inhibits protein synthesis by binding with the 30: and possibly the 50S ribosomal subunit(s) of susceptible bacteria; ma also cause alterations in the cytoplasmic membrane.
Adult Dosing 100 mg/day for 21 days or until improvement
Adjunctive treatment for periodontitis: 20 mg twice daily at least 1 hou before morning and evening meals for up to 9 months
Pregnancy Risk Factor D
Availability Rx

Doxycycline Hyclate

Common US Brand Names Vibramycin® Hyclate
Therapeutic Category Antibiotic, Tetracycline Derivative
Dosage Forms
Capsule
Tablet
Strength
Capsule: 50 mg, 100 mg
Periostat tablet: 20 mg
Tablet: 100 mg
How Supplied Desired quantity from stock
Manufacturer Numerous
Use in Oral Medicine Treatment of periodontitis associated with presenc of *Actinobacillus actinomycetemcomitans* (AA); principally in the treatmer of infections caused by susceptible *Rickettsia*, *Chlamydia*, and *Myco plasma* along with uncommon susceptible gram-negative an gram-positive organisms
Mechanism of Action Inhibits protein synthesis by binding with the 30S and possibly the 50S ribosomal subunit(s) of susceptible bacteria; ma also cause alterations in the cytoplasmic membrane.
Adult Dosing 100 mg/day for 21 days or until improvement
Adjunctive treatment for periodontitis: 20 mg twice daily at least 1 hou before morning and evening meals for up to 9 months
Pregnancy Risk Factor D
Availability Rx

♦ Evoxac™ see Cevimeline on page 137
♦ Flagyl® see Metronidazole on page 144

Fluconazole Tablets

Common US Brand Names Diflucan®
Therapeutic Category Antifungal Agent, Systemic
Dosage Forms Tablet
Strength 50 mg, 100 mg, 150 mg, 200 mg
How Supplied Desired quantity from stock
Manufacturer Pfizer
Use in Oral Medicine Oral fluconazole should be used in persons able t tolerate oral medications; parenteral fluconazole should be reserved fo patients who are both unable to take oral medications and are unable t tolerate amphotericin B (eg, due to hypersensitivity or renal insufficiency

Treatment of susceptible fungal infections in the oral cavity includin candidiasis, oral thrush, and chronic mucocutaneous candidiasis; treat ment of esophageal and oropharyngeal candidiasis caused by *Candid* species; treatment of severe, chronic mucocutaneous candidiasis cause by *Candida* species
Mechanism of Action Interferes with cytochrome P-450 activity decreasing ergosterol synthesis (principal sterol in fungal cell membrane and inhibiting cell membrane formation
Adult Dosing See table for once-daily dosing.

Indication	Day 1	Daily Therapy	Minimum Duration of Therapy
Oropharyngeal candidiasis	200 mg	100 mg	14 d
Esophageal candidiasis	200 mg	100 mg	21 d
Systemic candidiasis	400 mg	200 mg	28 d
Cryptococcal meningitis			10-12 wk after CSF culture becomes negative
acute	400 mg	200 mg	
relapse	200 mg	200 mg	

Pediatric Dosing Efficacy of fluconazole has not been established i children; a small number of patients from 3-13 years of age have beer treated with fluconazole using doses of 3-6 mg/kg/day once daily. Dose as high as 12 mg/kg/day once daily have been used to treat candidiasis i immunocompromised children; 10-12 mg/kg/day has been used prophy lactically against fungal infections in pediatric bone marrow transplar patients.

140

Pregnancy Risk Factor C
Availability Rx

Fluocinonide 0.05% (Ointment or Gel)

Common US Brand Names Lidex®
Therapeutic Category Corticosteroid, Topical (High Potency)
Ingredients
 Ointment: Active: Fluocinonide 0.5 mg/g; Other: Glyceryl monostearate, white petrolatum, propylene carbonate, propylene glycol, white wax
 Gel: Active: Fluocinonide 0.5mg/g; Other: Gel base consisting of carbomer 940, edetate disodium, propyl gallate, propylene glycol, sodium hydroxide and/or hydrochloric acid (to adjust the pH), and purified water
Dosage Forms Ointment, topical; Gel, topical
Strength 0.05%
How Supplied 15 g, 30 g, 60 g tubes ointment or gel
Manufacturer Medicis
Use in Oral Medicine Anti-inflammatory, antipruritic, relief of inflammatory and pruritic manifestations [high potency topical corticosteroid]
Mechanism of Action Not well defined for all topical corticosteroids; however, is felt to be a combination of three important properties: anti-inflammatory activity, immunosuppressive properties, and antiproliferative actions.
Adult Dosing Apply thin layer to affected area 2-4 times/day depending on the severity of the condition. Therapy should be discontinued when control is achieved; if no improvement is seen, reassessment of diagnosis may be necessary.
Pediatric Dosing Apply thin layer to affected area 2-4 times/day depending on the severity of the condition. Therapy should be discontinued when control is achieved; if no improvement is seen, reassessment of diagnosis may be necessary.
Pregnancy Risk Factor C
Availability Rx

Foscarnet

Common US Brand Names Foscavir®
Therapeutic Category Antiviral Agent, Parenteral
Dosage Forms Injectable
Strength 24 mg/mL
How Supplied 250 mL (12s); 500 mL (12s)
Manufacturer Astra Pharm
Use in Oral Medicine Approved indications in adult patients:
 Herpesvirus infections suspected to be caused by acyclovir (HSV, VZV) or ganciclovir (CMV) resistant strains (this occurs almost exclusively in persons with advanced AIDS who have received prolonged treatment for a herpesvirus infection)
 CMV retinitis in persons with AIDS
 Other CMV infections in persons unable to tolerate ganciclovir
Mechanism of Action Pyrophosphate analogue which acts as a noncompetitive inhibitor of many viral RNA and DNA polymerases as well as HIV reverse transcriptase. Inhibitory effects occur at concentrations which do not affect host cellular DNA polymerases; however, some human cell growth suppression has been observed with high *in vitro* concentrations. Similar to ganciclovir, foscarnet is a virostatic agent. Foscarnet does not require activation by thymidine kinase.
Adult Dosing Adolescents and Adults: I.V.:
 Induction treatment: 60 mg/kg/dose every 8 hours for 14-21 days
 Maintenance therapy: 90-120 mg/kg/day as a single infusion
 See tables.

Induction Dosing of Foscarnet in Patients with Abnormal Renal Function

Cl_{cr} (mL/min/kg)	HSV Equivalent to 40 mg/kg q12h	HSV Equivalent to 40 mg/kg q8h	CMV Equivalent to 60 mg/kg q8h	CMV Equivalent to 90 mg/kg q12h
<0.4	not recommended	not recommended	not recommended	not recommended
≥0.4-0.5	20 mg/kg every 24 hours	35 mg/kg every 24 hours	50 mg/kg every 24 hours	50 mg/kg every 24 hours
>0.5-0.6	25 mg/kg every 24 hours	40 mg/kg every 24 hours	60 mg/kg every 24 hours	60 mg/kg every 24 hours
>0.6-0.8	35 mg/kg every 24 hours	25 mg/kg every 12 hours	40 mg/kg every 12 hours	80 mg/kg every 24 hours
>0.8-1.0	20 mg/kg every 12 hours	35 mg/kg every 12 hours	50 mg/kg every 12 hours	50 mg/kg every 12 hours
>1.0-1.4	30 mg/kg every 12 hours	30 mg/kg every 8 hours	45 mg/kg every 8 hours	70 mg/kg every 12 hours
>1.4	40 mg/kg every 12 hours	40 mg/kg every 8 hours	60 mg/kg every 8 hours	90 mg/kg every 12 hours

Maintenance Dosing of Foscarnet in Patients with Abnormal Renal Function

Cl_{cr} (mL/min/kg)	CMV Equivalent to 90 mg/kg q24h	CMV Equivalent to 120 mg/kg q24h
<0.4	not recommended	not recommended
≥0.4-0.5	50 mg/kg every 48 hours	65 mg/kg every 48 hours
>0.5-0.6	60 mg/kg every 48 hours	80 mg/kg every 48 hours
>0.6-0.8	80 mg/kg every 48 hours	105 mg/kg every 48 hours
>0.8-1.0	50 mg/kg every 24 hours	65 mg/kg every 24 hours
>1.0-1.4	70 mg/kg every 24 hours	90 mg/kg every 24 hours
>1.4	90 mg/kg every 24 hours	120 mg/kg every 24 hours

Pregnancy Risk Factor C
Availability Rx

♦ Foscavir® *see* Foscarnet *on page 141*

♦ Fungizone® Cream 3% *see* Amphotericin B Cream 3% *on page 136*

Gabapentin

Common US Brand Names Neurontin®
Therapeutic Category Anticonvulsant, Miscellaneous
Dosage Forms
 Capsule
 Tablet
Strength
 Capsule: 100 mg, 300 mg, 400 mg
 Tablet: 600 mg, 800 mg
How Supplied Desired quantity from stock
Manufacturer Various
Use in Oral Medicine Neuropathic pain in consult with physician
Mechanism of Action Exact mechanism of action is not known, but does have properties in common with other anticonvulsants; although structurally related to GABA, it does not interact with GABA receptors
Adult Dosing 300 mg 3-5 times/day
Pregnancy Risk Factor C
Availability Rx

♦ Generic only *see* Nystatin/Triamcinolone Acetate Ointment *on page 145*

♦ Gengraf® *see* Cyclosporine *on page 139*

Ibuprofen OTC

Common US Brand Names Advil®; Motrin IB®
Therapeutic Category Analgesic, Non-narcotic; Anti-inflammatory Agent; Nonsteroidal Anti-inflammatory Drug (NSAID), Oral
Dosage Forms
 Suspension, oral
 Tablet
 Tablet, chewable
Strength
 Suspension, oral: 100 mg/5 mL
 Tablet: 200 mg
 Tablet, chewable: 50 mg, 100 mg
How Supplied Various commercial package sizes
Manufacturer Numerous
Use in Oral Medicine Management of pain and swelling
Mechanism of Action Inhibits prostaglandin synthesis by decreasing the activity of the enzyme, cyclo-oxygenase, which results in decreased formation of prostaglandin precursors
Adult Dosing 400-800 mg/dose 3-4 times/day
Maximum Adult Dose Maximum daily dose: 3.2 (3200 mg) g/day
Pediatric Dosing Analgesic: 4-10 mg/kg/dose every 6-8 hours
Pregnancy Risk Factor B (D in third trimester)
Availability OTC
Comment Preoperative use of ibuprofen at a dose of 400-600 mg every 6 hours 24 hours before the appointment decreases postoperative edema and hastens healing time

Imiquimod

Common US Brand Names Aldara™
Therapeutic Category Immune Response Modifier
Ingredients Active: Imiquimod 50 mg/g; Other: Vanishing cream base consisting of isostearic acid, cetyl alcohol, stearyl alcohol, white petrolatum, polysorbate 60, sorbitan monostearate, glycerin, xanthine gum, purified water, benzyl alcohol, methylparaben, propylparaben
Dosage Forms Cream
Strength 5%
(Continued)

Imiquimod (Continued)

How Supplied 5%, 250 mg (12s)
Manufacturer 3M Pharm
Use in Oral Medicine Oral, genital, and perianal warts (condyloma acuminata)
Mechanism of Action Mechanism of action is unknown; however, induces cytokines, including interferon-alfa and others
Adult Dosing Topical: Apply 3 times/week, prior to bedtime, leave on for 6-10 hours, remove cream by washing area with mild soap and water
Pregnancy Risk Factor B
Availability Rx

♦ Imuran® see Azathioprine on page 136

Interferon Alfa-2b

Common US Brand Names Intron® A
Therapeutic Category Antineoplastic Agent, Miscellaneous; Biological Response Modulator; Interferon
Dosage Forms Powder for injection
Strength 3, 5, 10, 18, 25, 50 million int. units
How Supplied Powder for injection with diluent in vial
Manufacturer Schering
Use in Oral Medicine
Patients >1 year of age: Chronic hepatitis B
Patients >18 years of age: Condyloma acuminata, chronic hepatitis C, hairy cell leukemia, malignant melanoma, AIDS-related Kaposi's sarcoma, follicular non-Hodgkin's lymphoma
Mechanism of Action Alfa interferons are a family of proteins, produced by nucleated cells, that have antiviral, antiproliferative, and immune-regulating activity. There are 16 known subtypes of alpha interferons. Interferons interact with cells through high affinity cell surface receptors. Following activation, multiple effects can be detected including induction of gene transcription. Inhibits cellular growth, alters the state of cellular differentiation, interferes with oncogene expression, alters cell surface antigen expression, increases phagocytic activity of macrophages, and augments cytotoxicity of lymphocytes for target cells
Adult Dosing Refer to individual protocols:
Hairy cell leukemia: I.M., S.C.: 2 million units/m^2 3 times/week for 2 to ≥6 months of therapy
AIDS-related Kaposi's sarcoma: I.M., S.C. (use 50 million unit vial): 30 million units/m^2 3 times/week
Condylomata acuminata: Intralesionally (use 10 million unit vial): 1 million units/lesion 3 times/week for 4-8 weeks; not to exceed 5 million units per treatment (maximum: 5 lesions at one time)
Chronic hepatitis C (non-A/non-B): I.M., S.C.: 3 million units 3 times/week for approximately a 6-month course
Chronic hepatitis B: I.M., S.C.: 5 million units/day or 10 million units 3 times/week for 16 weeks; if severe adverse reactions occur, reduce dosage 50% or temporarily discontinue therapy until adverse reactions abate; when platelet/granulocyte count returns to normal, reinstitute therapy
Pregnancy Risk Factor C
Availability Rx

♦ Intron® A see Interferon Alfa-2b on page 142

Iodoquinol and Hydrocortisone

Common US Brand Names Vytone®
Therapeutic Category Antifungal Agent, Topical; Corticosteroid, Topical
Dosage Forms Cream
Strength 1% - 1%
How Supplied 30 g tube
Manufacturer Dermik
Use in Oral Medicine Treatment of angular cheilitis
Adult Dosing Apply 3-4 times/day
Pregnancy Risk Factor C
Availability Rx

Itraconazole Capsules

Common US Brand Names Sporanox®
Therapeutic Category Antifungal Agent, Systemic
Dosage Forms Capsule
Strength 100 mg
How Supplied 28s ea, 30s ea of 100 mg capsules
Manufacturer Janssen
Use in Oral Medicine Treatment of susceptible fungal infections in immunocompromised and immunocompetent patients including blastomycosis and histoplasmosis; also has activity against *Aspergillus, Candida, Coccidioides, Cryptococcus, Sporothrix* and chromomycosis

Useful in superficial mycoses including dermatophytoses (eg, tinea capitis), pityriasis versicolor, sebopsoriasis, vaginal and chronic mucocutaneous candidiases; systemic mycoses including candidiasis, meningeal and disseminated cryptococcal infections, paracoccidioidomycosis, coccidioidomycoses; miscellaneous mycoses such as sporotrichosis, chromomycosis, leishmaniasis, fungal keratitis, alternariosis, zygomycosis
Mechanism of Action Inhibits fungal cytochrome P-450-dependent enzymes (CYP3A4 and CYP2C); this blocks the synthesis of ergosterol which is the vital component in the fungal cell membrane. Triazoles contain three nitrogen atoms in the five-membered azole ring; the triazole ring increases tissue penetration, prolongs half-life, and enhances efficacy while decreasing toxicity compared with the imidazoles.
Adult Dosing Oral (absorption is best if taken with food, therefore, it is best to administer itraconazole after meals): 200 mg once daily, if obvious improvement or there is evidence of progressive fungal disease, increase the dose in 100 mg increments; doses >200 mg/day are given in 2 divided doses
Maximum Adult Dose 400 mg/day
Pediatric Dosing Oral (absorption is best if taken with food, therefore, it is best to administer itraconazole after meals): Efficacy and safety have not been established; a small number of patients 3-16 years of age have been treated with 100 mg/day for systemic fungal infections with no serious adverse effects reported
Pregnancy Risk Factor C
Availability Rx

♦ Kaopectate® see Attapulgite Suspension on page 136

♦ Keflex® see Cephalexin on page 137

♦ Kenalog® in Orabase® see Triamcinolone Acetate in Orabase® on page 146

♦ Kenalog® Ointment see Triamcinolone Ointment on page 146

Ketoconazole Cream 2%

Common US Brand Names Nizoral®
Therapeutic Category Antifungal Agent, Topical
Ingredients Active: Ketoconazole 2%; Other: Aqueous cream vehicle consisting of propylene glycol, stearyl and cetyl alcohols, sorbitan mono-stearate, polysorbate 60, isopropyl myristate, sodium sulfite anhydrous, polysorbate 80, purified water
Dosage Forms Cream, topical
Strength 2%
How Supplied 15 g, 30 g, 60 g tubes
Manufacturer Numerous
Use in Oral Medicine Treatment of susceptible fungal infections in the oral cavity including candidiasis, oral thrush, and chronic mucocutaneous candidiasis
Mechanism of Action Alters the permeability of the cell wall; inhibits biosynthesis of triglycerides and phospholipids by fungi; inhibits several fungal enzymes that results in a build-up of toxic concentrations of hydrogen peroxide
Adult Dosing Rub gently into the affected area once daily to twice daily
Pregnancy Risk Factor C
Availability Rx

Ketoconazole Tablets

Common US Brand Names Nizoral®
Therapeutic Category Antifungal Agent, Systemic
Dosage Forms Tablet
Strength 200 mg
How Supplied 200 mg tablets
Manufacturer Numerous
Use in Oral Medicine Treatment of susceptible fungal infections in the oral cavity including candidiasis, oral thrush, and chronic mucocutaneous candidiasis
Mechanism of Action Alters the permeability of the cell wall; inhibits biosynthesis of triglycerides and phospholipids by fungi; inhibits several fungal enzymes that results in a build-up of toxic concentrations of hydrogen peroxide
Adult Dosing Adults: 200-400 mg/day as a single daily dose for for 1-2 weeks for candidiasis, for at least 4 weeks in recalcitrant dermatophyte infections, and for up to 6 months for other systemic mycoses
Pediatric Dosing ≥2 years: 3.3-6.6 mg/kg/day as a single dose for 1-2 weeks for candidiasis, for at least 4 weeks in recalcitrant dermatophyte infections, and for up to 6 months for other systemic mycoses
Pregnancy Risk Factor C
Availability Rx

♦ Klonopin® see Clonazepam on page 138

♦ Lactinex® see Lactobacillus acidophilus and Lactobacillus bulgaricus on page 143

Lactobacillus acidophilus and *Lactobacillus bulgaricus*

Common US Brand Names Bacid®; Lactinex®
Therapeutic Category Antidiarrheal
Dosage Forms
Capsule
Granules
Powder
Tablet
How Supplied
Powder: 1 g/packet (144s)
Tablet: 12x50 (600s)
Manufacturer BD Microbiology
Use in Oral Medicine Treatment of uncomplicated diarrhea particularly that caused by antibiotic therapy; re-establish normal physiologic and bacterial flora of the intestinal tract
Mechanism of Action Creates an environment unfavorable to potentially pathogenic fungi or bacteria through the production of lactic acid, and favors establishment of an aciduric flora, thereby suppressing the growth of pathogenic microorganisms; helps re-establish normal intestinal flora
Adult Dosing
Capsules: 2 capsules 2-4 times/day
Granules: 1 packet added to or taken with cereal, food, milk, fruit juice, or water, 3-4 times/day
Powder: 1 teaspoonful daily with liquid
Tablet, chewable: 4 tablets 3-4 times/day; may follow each dose with a small amount of milk, fruit juice, or water
Pediatric Dosing Children >3 years:
Capsules: 2 capsules 2-4 times/day
Granules: 1 packet added to or taken with cereal, food, milk, fruit juice, or water, 3-4 times/day
Powder: 1 teaspoonful daily with liquid
Tablet, chewable: 4 tablets 3-4 times/day; may follow each dose with a small amount of milk, fruit juice, or water
Availability OTC

♦ Lidex® *see* Fluocinonide 0.05% (Ointment or Gel) *on page 141*

Lidocaine Viscous 2%

Common US Brand Names Xylocaine®
Therapeutic Category Dental/Local Anesthetics
Dosage Forms Solution
Strength 2% lidocaine
How Supplied 100 mL
Manufacturer Astra Pharm LP
Use in Oral Medicine Topical local anesthetic to give supportive care for some oral ulcers
Mechanism of Action Blocks both the initiation and conduction of nerve impulses by decreasing the neuronal membrane's permeability to sodium ions, which results in inhibition of depolarization with resultant blockade of conduction
Maximum Adult Dose Do not exceed 6.6 mg/kg of body weight or 300 mg/dental appointment.

Note: Maximum dose for lidocaine hydrochloride cited from USP Dispensing Information (USP DI) 17th ed, The United Pharmacopeial Convention, Inc, Rockville, MD, 1997, 137.
Pregnancy Risk Factor C
Availability Rx
Comment Patient should be advised not to swallow; may alter gag reflex

♦ Listerine® Antiseptic *see* Antiseptic Mouth Rinse *on page 136*

Lysine Tablets

Common US Brand Names Lysinyl®
Therapeutic Category Dietary Supplement
Dosage Forms Tablets; Capsules
Strength
Capsule: 500 mg
Tablet: 500 mg, 1000 mg
How Supplied 500 mg (100s ea); 1000 mg (60s ea, 100s ea)
Manufacturer Numerous
Use in Oral Medicine Improves utilization of vegetable proteins
Adult Dosing 334-1500 mg/day
Pregnancy Risk Factor C
Availability OTC

♦ Lysinyl® *see* Lysine Tablets *on page 143*

♦ Maalox® *see* Magnesium Hydroxide / Aluminum Hydroxide Suspension *on page 143*

Magnesium Hydroxide / Aluminum Hydroxide Suspension

Common US Brand Names Maalox®
Therapeutic Category Antacid
Dosage Forms Suspension
Strength Magnesium hydroxide: 200 mg/5 mL; aluminum hydroxide: 225 mg/5 mL
How Supplied
Maalox® Cooling Mint: 5 oz, 12 oz
Maalox® Smooth Cherry: 12 oz, 26 oz
Maalox® Refreshing Lemon: 12 oz, 26 oz
Manufacturer Novartis
Use in Oral Medicine Sometimes used as a coating agent in combination with Benadryl® for treatment of oral ulcers
Adult Dosing Mix 50:50 with Benadryl® elixir for topical application
Pregnancy Risk Factor C
Availability OTC
Comment Sodium content of 5 mL (Maalox®): 1.3 mg (0.06 mEq)

♦ Medrol® Dose Pack *see* Methylprednisolone *on page 143*

Methotrexate

Common US Brand Names Rheumatrex®; Trexall™
Therapeutic Category Antineoplastic Agent, Antimetabolite
Dosage Forms
Powder for reconstitution
Solution for injection
Tablet
Strength
Injection, powder for reconstitution [preservative free]: 20 mg, 1 g
Injection, solution, as sodium: 25 mg/mL (2 mL, 10 mL) [contains benzyl alcohol]
Injection, solution, as sodium [preservative free]: 25 mg/mL (2 mL, 4 mL, 8 mL, 10 mL)
Tablet, as sodium: 2.5 mg
Rheumatrex®: 2.5 mg
Trexall™: 5 mg, 7.5 mg, 10 mg, 15 mg
Tablet, as sodium [dose pack] (Rheumatrex® Dose Pack): 2.5 mg (4 cards with 2, 3, 4, 5, or 6 tablets each)
How Supplied Desired quantity from stock
Manufacturer Various
Use in Oral Medicine Soft tissue sarcomas
Mechanism of Action Methotrexate is a folate antimetabolite that inhibits DNA synthesis. Methotrexate irreversibly binds to dihydrofolate reductase, inhibiting the formation of reduced folates, and thymidylate synthetase, resulting in inhibition of purine and thymidylic acid synthesis. Methotrexate is cell cycle specific for the S phase of the cycle.
Adult Dosing Refer to individual protocols.
Note: Doses between 100 mg/m^2 to 500 mg/m^2 may require leucovorin rescue. Doses >500 mg/m^2 require leucovorin rescue.
Antineoplastic dosage range: I.V.: Range is wide from 30-40 mg/m^2/week to 100-12,000 mg/m^2 with leucovorin rescue
Sarcoma: I.V.: 8-12 g/m^2 weekly for 2-4 weeks
Pregnancy Risk Factor X (psoriasis, rheumatoid arthritis)
Availability Rx

Methylprednisolone

Common US Brand Names Medrol® Dose Pack
Therapeutic Category Adrenal Corticosteroid; Anti-inflammatory Agent; Corticosteroid, Systemic; Corticosteroid, Topical (Low Potency)
Dosage Forms Tablet
Strength 4 mg
How Supplied Package of 21 tablets
Manufacturer Pharmacia/Upjohn
Use in Oral Medicine Treatment of a variety of oral diseases of allergic, inflammatory, or autoimmune origin
Mechanism of Action Decreases inflammation by suppression of migration of polymorphonuclear leukocytes and reversal of increased capillary permeability
Adult Dosing Anti-inflammatory or immunosuppressive: 2-60 mg/day in 1-4 divided doses to start, followed by gradual reduction in dosage to the lowest possible level consistent with maintaining an adequate clinical response. Therapy should be discontinued when control is achieved; if no improvement is seen, reassessment of diagnosis may be necessary.
Pediatric Dosing Anti-inflammatory or immunosuppressive: 0.5-1.7 mg/kg/day or 5-25 mg/m^2/day in divided doses every 6-12 hours. Therapy should be discontinued when control is achieved; if no improvement is seen, reassessment of diagnosis may be necessary.
Pregnancy Risk Factor C
Availability Rx

♦ Meticorten® *see* Prednisone *on page 145*

Metronidazole

Common US Brand Names Flagyl®
Therapeutic Category Amebicide; Antibiotic, Anaerobic; Antiprotozoal
Dosage Forms Tablet
Strength 250 mg, 500 mg
How Supplied Desired quantity from stock
Manufacturer Numerous
Use in Oral Medicine Treatment of oral soft tissue infections due to anaerobic bacteria including all anaerobic cocci, anaerobic gram-negative bacilli (*Bacteroides*), and gram-positive spore-forming bacilli (*Clostridium*). Useful as single agent or in combination with amoxicillin, Augmentin®, or ciprofloxacin in the treatment of periodontitis associated with the presence of *Actinobacillus actinomycetemcomitans*, (AA).
Mechanism of Action Reduced to a product which interacts with DNA to cause a loss of helical DNA structure and strand breakage resulting in inhibition of protein synthesis and cell death in susceptible organisms
Adult Dosing
Anaerobic infections: 500 mg every 6-8 hours
Treatment of periodontitis associated with AA:
Oral, singly: 200-400 mg 3 times/day for 7-10 days;
In combination: Metronidazole plus Augmentin® 250 mg 3 times/day each for 7 days; metronidazole 250 mg plus amoxicillin 250 mg each 3 times/day for 7 days; metronidazole plus ciprofloxacin 500 mg each twice daily for 8 days
Maximum Adult Dose Anaerobic infections: Not to exceed 4 g/day
Pregnancy Risk Factor B
Availability Rx

♦ Motrin IB® *see* Ibuprofen OTC *on page 141*

♦ Mycelex® *see* Clotrimazole Oral Troche *on page 138*

♦ Mycostatin® *see* Nystatin Oral Suspension *on page 144*

♦ Naprosyn® *see* Naproxen *on page 144*

Naproxen

Common US Brand Names Naprosyn®
Therapeutic Category Analgesic, Non-narcotic; Anti-inflammatory Agent; Nonsteroidal Anti-inflammatory Drug (NSAID), Oral
Dosage Forms
Suspension, oral
Tablet
Tablet, delayed release
Strength
Suspension, oral: 125 mg/5 mL
Tablet: 250 mg, 375 mg, 500 mg
Tablet, delayed release: 375 mg, 500 mg
How Supplied
Suspension, oral: 1 pint bottles
Tablet, delayed-release: Desired quantity from stock
Manufacturer Roche Pharmaceuticals
Use in Oral Medicine Management of pain and swelling
Mechanism of Action Inhibits prostaglandin synthesis by decreasing the activity of the enzyme, cyclo-oxygenase, which results in decreased formation of prostaglandin precursors
Adult Dosing Initial: 500 mg, then 250 mg every 6-8 hours
Maximum Adult Dose 1250 mg/day naproxen base
Pregnancy Risk Factor B (D in third trimester)
Availability Rx
Comment The sodium salt of naproxen provides better effects because of better oral absorption; the sodium salt also provides a faster onset and a longer duration of action

Naproxen Sodium

Common US Brand Names Anaprox®; Anaprox DS®
Therapeutic Category Analgesic, Non-narcotic; Anti-inflammatory Agent; Nonsteroidal Anti-inflammatory Drug (NSAID), Oral
Dosage Forms Tablet
Strength 275 mg, 550 mg
How Supplied Desired quantity from stock
Manufacturer Roche Pharmaceuticals
Use in Oral Medicine Management of pain and swelling
Mechanism of Action Inhibits prostaglandin synthesis by decreasing the activity of the enzyme, cyclo-oxygenase, which results in decreased formation of prostaglandin precursors
Adult Dosing Initial: 550 mg, then 275 mg every 6-8 hours
Maximum Adult Dose 1375 mg/day naproxen sodium
Pregnancy Risk Factor B (D in third trimester)
Availability Rx

Comment The sodium salt of naproxen provides better effects because better oral absorption; the sodium salt also provides a faster onset and longer duration of action

Naproxen Sodium OTC

Common US Brand Names Aleve®
Therapeutic Category Analgesic, Non-narcotic; Anti-inflammatory Agent; Nonsteroidal Anti-inflammatory Drug (NSAID), Oral
Dosage Forms Caplet, gelcap, tablet
Strength 220 mg
How Supplied Various commercial package sizes
Manufacturer Numerous
Use in Oral Medicine Management of pain and swelling
Mechanism of Action Inhibits prostaglandin synthesis by decreasing the activity of the enzyme, cyclo-oxygenase, which results in decreased formation of prostaglandin precursors
Adult Dosing Initial: 550 mg, then 275 mg every 6-8 hours
Maximum Adult Dose 1375 mg/day naproxen sodium
Pregnancy Risk Factor B (D in third trimester)
Availability OTC
Comment The sodium salt of naproxen provides better effects because better oral absorption; the sodium salt also provides a faster onset and longer duration of action

♦ Neoral® *see* Cyclosporine *on page 139*

♦ Neurontin® *see* Gabapentin *on page 141*

♦ Nizoral® *see* Ketoconazole Cream 2% *on page 142*

♦ Nizoral® *see* Ketoconazole Tablets *on page 142*

Nortriptyline

Common US Brand Names Pamelor®
Therapeutic Category Antidepressant, Tricyclic (Secondary Amine)
Dosage Forms
Capsule
Solution
Strength
Capsule: 10 mg, 25 mg, 50 mg, 75 mg
Solution: 10 mg/5 mL
How Supplied Desired quantity from stock
Manufacturer Various
Use in Oral Medicine Treatment of burning mouth syndrome and neuropathic pain
Mechanism of Action Traditionally believed to increase the synaptic concentration of serotonin and/or norepinephrine in the central nervous system by inhibition of their reuptake by the presynaptic neuronal membrane. However, additional receptor effects have been found including desensitization of adenyl cyclase, down regulation of beta-adrenergic receptors, and down regulation of serotonin receptors.
Adult Dosing 10-50 mg/day
Pregnancy Risk Factor D
Availability Rx

Nystatin Oral Suspension

Common US Brand Names Mycostatin®
Therapeutic Category Antifungal Agent, Oral Nonabsorbed
Ingredients Unavailable
Dosage Forms Suspension, oral
Strength 100,000 units/mL
How Supplied 60 mL, 480 mL
Manufacturer Apothecon
Use in Oral Medicine Treatment of susceptible cutaneous, mucocutaneous, and oral cavity fungal infections normally caused by the *Candida* species
Mechanism of Action Binds to sterols in fungal cell membrane, changing the cell wall permeability allowing for leakage of cellular contents
Adult Dosing Oral candidiasis: Suspension (swish and swallow orally) 400,000-600,000 units 4 times/day
Pediatric Dosing Oral candidiasis: Suspension (swish and swallow orally) 400,000-600,000 units 4 times/day
Pregnancy Risk Factor C
Availability Rx

Nystatin Topical

Therapeutic Category Antifungal Agent, Topical
Ingredients Unavailable
Dosage Forms
Cream, topical
Ointment, topical

Strength 100,000 units per g
How Supplied 15 g; 30 g tubes
Manufacturer Numerous
Use in Oral Medicine Treatment of susceptible cutaneous, mucocutaneous, and oral cavity fungal infections normally caused by the *Candida* species
Mechanism of Action Binds to sterols in fungal cell membrane, changing the cell wall permeability allowing for leakage of cellular contents
Adult Dosing 400,000-600,000 units 4 times/day
Pediatric Dosing 400,000-600,000 units 4 times/day
Pregnancy Risk Factor B
Availability Rx

Nystatin/Triamcinolone Acetate Ointment

Common US Brand Names Generic only
Therapeutic Category Antifungal Agent, Topical; Corticosteroid, Topical (Medium Potency)
Ingredients Unavailable
Dosage Forms Ointment, topical
Strength 100,000 units nystatin / 0.1% triamcinolone
How Supplied 15 g, 30 g, 60 g tubes
Manufacturer Apothecon
Use in Oral Medicine Treatment of angular cheilitis and cutaneous candidiasis
Mechanism of Action Nystatin is an antifungal agent that binds to sterols in fungal cell membrane, changing the cell wall permeability allowing for leakage of cellular contents. Triamcinolone is a synthetic corticosteroid; it decreases inflammation by suppression of migration of polymorphonuclear leukocytes and reversal of increased capillary permeability. It suppresses the immune system reducing activity and volume of the lymphatic system. It suppresses adrenal function at high doses.
Adult Dosing Apply sparingly 2-4 times/day; therapy should be discontinued when control is achieved; if no improvement is seen, reassessment of diagnosis may be necessary.
Pediatric Dosing Apply sparingly 2-4 times/day; therapy should be discontinued when control is achieved; if no improvement is seen, reassessment of diagnosis may be necessary.
Pregnancy Risk Factor C
Availability Rx

♦ Orabase®-B *see* Benzocaine Paste *on page 137*

♦ Orabase®-B Maximum Strength *see* Benzocaine Gel *on page 137*

♦ Pamelor® *see* Nortriptyline *on page 144*

Penciclovir Cream

Common US Brand Names Denavir™ Cream
Therapeutic Category Antiviral Agent, Topical
Ingredients Active: Penciclovir 10 mg/g; Other: Cetomacrogol 1000 BP, cetostearyl alcohol, mineral oil, propylene glycol, purified water, white petrolatum
Dosage Forms Cream, topical
Strength 1%
How Supplied 2 g tube
Manufacturer SK Beecham
Use in Oral Medicine Antiviral cream for the treatment of recurrent herpes labialis (cold sores) in adults
Mechanism of Action In cells infected with HSV-1 or HSV-2, viral thymidine kinase phosphorylates penciclovir to a monophosphate form which, in turn, is converted to penciclovir triphosphate by cellular kinases. Penciclovir triphosphate inhibits HSV polymerase competitively with deoxyguanosine triphosphate. Consequently, herpes viral DNA synthesis and, therefore, replication are selectively inhibited
Adult Dosing Apply cream at the first sign or symptom of cold sore (eg, tingling, swelling); apply every 2 hours during waking hours for 4 days
Pregnancy Risk Factor B
Availability Rx

Penicillin V Potassium

Common US Brand Names Pen.Vee® K; V-Cillin K®; Veetids®
Therapeutic Category Antibiotic, Penicillin
Dosage Forms
  Powder for oral solution
  Tablet
Strength
  Powder: 125 mg/5 mL, 250 mg/5 mL
  Tablet: 250 mg, 500 mg
How Supplied
  Powder (when reconstituted): 100 mL, 200 mL
  Tablets: Desired quantity from stock

Manufacturer Numerous
Use in Oral Medicine Antibiotic of first choice in treating common orofacial infections caused by aerobic gram-positive cocci and anaerobes. These orofacial infections include cellulitis, periapical abscess, periodontal abscess, acute suppurative pulpitis, oronasal fistula, pericoronitis, osteitis, osteomyelitis, postsurgical and post-traumatic infection. It is no longer recommended for dental procedure prophylaxis.
Mechanism of Action Inhibits bacterial cell wall synthesis by binding to one or more of the penicillin binding proteins (PBPs); which in turn inhibits the final transpeptidation step of peptidoglycan synthesis in bacterial cell walls, thus inhibiting cell wall biosynthesis. Bacteria eventually lyse due to ongoing activity of cell wall autolytic enzymes (autolysins and murein hydrolases) while cell wall assembly is arrested.
Adult Dosing Children >12 years and Adults: 250-500 mg every 6 hours for at least 7 days
Pediatric Dosing <12 years: Daily dose: 25-50 mg/kg in divided doses every 6-8 hours for 7 days
Maximum Child Dose 3 g/day
Pregnancy Risk Factor B
Availability Rx

♦ Pen.Vee® K *see* Penicillin V Potassium *on page 145*

♦ Peridex® *see* Chlorhexidine Gluconate *on page 138*

♦ PerioGard® *see* Chlorhexidine Gluconate *on page 138*

Pilocarpine Oral

Common US Brand Names Salagen®
Therapeutic Category Cholinergic Agent
Dosage Forms Tablet
Strength 5 mg
How Supplied Desired quantity from stock
Manufacturer MGI
Use in Oral Medicine Treatment of xerostomia caused by radiation therapy in patients with head and neck cancer and from Sjögren's syndrome
Mechanism of Action Pilocarpine stimulates the muscarinic-type acetylcholine receptors in the salivary glands within the parasympathetic division of the autonomic nervous system to cause an increase in serous-type saliva
Adult Dosing 1-2 tablets 3-4 times/day; patients should be treated for a minimum of 90 days for optimum effects
Maximum Adult Dose 30 mg/day
Pregnancy Risk Factor C
Availability Rx

Prednisone

Common US Brand Names Deltasone®; Meticorten®
Therapeutic Category Adrenal Corticosteroid; Anti-inflammatory Agent; Corticosteroid, Systemic
Dosage Forms Tablet
Strength 5 mg, 10 mg, 20 mg, 50 mg
How Supplied Desired quantity from stock
Manufacturer Numerous
Use in Oral Medicine Treatment of a variety of oral diseases of allergic, inflammatory or autoimmune origin
Mechanism of Action Decreases inflammation by suppression of migration of polymorphonuclear leukocytes and reversal of increased capillary permeability; suppresses the immune system by reducing activity and volume of the lymphatic system; suppresses adrenal function at high doses
Adult Dosing Dose depends upon condition being treated and response of patient; dosage for infants and children should be based on severity of the disease and response of the patient rather than on strict adherence to dosage indicated by age, weight, or body surface area. Consider alternate day therapy for long-term therapy. Discontinuation of long-term therapy requires gradual withdrawal by tapering the dose.
  Adults: 5-60 mg/day in divided doses 1-4 times/day
  Elderly: Use the lowest effective dose
Pediatric Dosing Dose depends upon condition being treated and response of patient; dosage for infants and children should be based on severity of the disease and response of the patient rather than on strict adherence to dosage indicated by age, weight, or body surface area. Consider alternate day therapy for long-term therapy. Discontinuation of long-term therapy requires gradual withdrawal by tapering the dose.
  Anti-inflammatory or immunosuppressive dose: 0.05-2 mg/kg/day divided 1-4 times/day
Pregnancy Risk Factor B
Availability Rx

♦ Restasis™ *see* Cyclosporine *on page 139*

♦ Rheumatrex® *see* Methotrexate *on page 143*

♦ Salagen® *see* Pilocarpine Oral *on page 145*

♦ Sandimmune® *see* Cyclosporine *on page 139*

♦ Sinequan® *see* Doxepin *on page 140*

♦ Sporanox® *see* Itraconazole Capsules *on page 142*

♦ Sumycin® *see* Tetracycline Syrup (125 mg/5 mL) *on page 146*

Tacrolimus

Therapeutic Category Immunosuppressant Agent; Topical Skin Product
Dosage Forms Ointment, topical
Strength 0.03%, 0.1%
How Supplied 0.03%: 30 g, 60 g, 100 g tubes; 0.1%: 30 g, 60 g, 100 g tubes
Manufacturer Fujisawa
Use in Oral Medicine Topical agent for treatment of severe ulcerative or vesiculobullous lesions, usually in consult with patient's physician
Mechanism of Action Suppresses cellular immunity (inhibits T-lymphocyte activation), possibly by binding to an intracellular protein, FKBP-12
Adult Dosing Atopic dermatitis (moderate to severe): Topical: Apply 0.03% or 0.1% ointment to affected area twice daily; rub in gently and completely; continue applications for 1 week after symptoms have cleared
Pregnancy Risk Factor C
Availability Rx

♦ Temovate® *see* Clobetasol Propionate Ointment 0.05% *on page 138*

Tetracycline Syrup (125 mg/5 mL)

Common US Brand Names Sumycin®
Therapeutic Category Antibiotic, Tetracycline Derivative
Dosage Forms Suspension, oral
Strength 125 mg/5 mL
How Supplied Desired quantity from stock
Manufacturer Numerous
Use in Oral Medicine Treatment of periodontitis associated with presence of *Actinobacillus actinomycetemcomitans* (AA); as adjunctive therapy in recurrent aphthous ulcers
Mechanism of Action Inhibits bacterial protein synthesis by binding with the 30S and possibly the 50S ribosomal subunit(s) of susceptible bacteria; may also cause alterations in the cytoplasmic membrane
Adult Dosing 250 mg every 6 hours until improvement (usually 10 days or more)
Pregnancy Risk Factor D
Availability Rx

♦ Trexall™ *see* Methotrexate *on page 143*

Triamcinolone Acetate in Orabase®

Common US Brand Names Kenalog® in Orabase®
Therapeutic Category Anti-inflammatory Agent
Ingredients Unavailable
Dosage Forms Paste
Strength 0.1%
How Supplied 5 g tube
Manufacturer Apothecon
Use in Oral Medicine For adjunctive treatment and for the temporary relief of symptoms associated with oral inflammatory lesions and ulcerative lesions
Mechanism of Action Decreases inflammation by suppression of migration of polymorphonuclear leukocytes and reversal of increased capillary permeability; suppresses the immune system by reducing activity and volume of the lymphatic system; suppresses adrenal function at high doses

Adult Dosing Press a small dab (about ¼ inch) to the lesion until a thin film develops. A larger quantity may be required for coverage of some lesions. For optimal results use only enough to coat the lesion with a thin film.
Pregnancy Risk Factor C
Availability Rx

Triamcinolone Ointment

Common US Brand Names Kenalog® Ointment
Therapeutic Category Anti-inflammatory Agent; Corticosteroid, Topical (Medium Potency)
Ingredients Unavailable
Dosage Forms Ointment
Strength 0.1%, 15 g, 80 g; 0.025%, 15 g
How Supplied 15 g, 80 g tube
Manufacturer Various
Use in Oral Medicine Management of mild to moderate ulcers, swelling or immunosuppression
Mechanism of Action Decreases inflammation by suppression of migration of polymorphonuclear leukocytes and reversal of increased capillary permeability; suppresses the immune system by reducing activity and volume of the lymphatic system; suppresses adrenal function at high doses
Adult Dosing Children >12 years and Adults: Topical: Apply a thin film 2 times/day; therapy should be discontinued when control is achieved; if no improvement is seen, reassessment of diagnosis may be necessary.
Pregnancy Risk Factor C
Availability Rx

♦ Trimox® *see* Amoxicillin *on page 135*

♦ Tylenol® *see* Acetaminophen *on page 134*

Valacyclovir

Common US Brand Names Valtrex®
Therapeutic Category Antiviral Agent, Oral
Dosage Forms Caplet
Strength 500 mg, 1000 mg
How Supplied Desired quantity from stock
Manufacturer Various
Use in Oral Medicine Treatment of recurrent herpes labialis and herpes zoster
Mechanism of Action Valacyclovir is rapidly and nearly completely converted to acyclovir by intestinal and hepatic metabolism. Acyclovir converted to acyclovir monophosphate by virus-specific thymidine kinase, then further converted to acyclovir triphosphate by other cellular enzymes. Acyclovir triphosphate inhibits DNA synthesis and viral replication by competing with deoxyguanosine triphosphate for viral DNA polymerase and being incorporated into viral DNA.
Adult Dosing
Recurrent herpes labialis: 2 g twice daily in 2 doses 12 hours apart
Herpes zoster: 1 g 3 times/day for 7 days
Pregnancy Risk Factor B
Availability Rx

♦ Valtrex® *see* Valacyclovir *on page 146*

♦ V-Cillin K® *see* Penicillin V Potassium *on page 145*

♦ Veetids® *see* Penicillin V Potassium *on page 145*

♦ Vibramycin® Hyclate *see* Doxycycline Hyclate *on page 140*

♦ Vibramycin® Syrup *see* Doxycycline Calcium Syrup *on page 140*

♦ Vytone® *see* Iodoquinol and Hydrocortisone *on page 142*

♦ Xylocaine® *see* Lidocaine Viscous 2% *on page 143*

♦ Zonalon® *see* Doxepin *on page 140*

♦ Zovirax® *see* Acyclovir Oral (Capsules or Tablets) *on page 134*

♦ Zovirax® *see* Acyclovir Topical *on page 134*

EXAMPLE PRESCRIPTIONS

These prescriptions are a limited, selected reference for the practitioner. More inclusive therapeutically-indexed drugs can be found in the current edition of Wynn RL, Meiller TF, and Crossley HL, *Drug Information Handbook for Dentistry*, Hudson, OH: Lexi-Comp, Inc.

PAIN MANAGEMENT

OVER-THE-COUNTER PRESCRIPTION EXAMPLES

Rx

Aspirin 325 mg
Disp
Sig: Take 2-3 tablets every 4 hours

Rx

Ibuprofen 200 mg
Disp
Sig: Take 2-3 tablets every 4 hours, up to
  3200 mg (16 tablets)/day

Note: Ibuprofen is available over-the-counter as Motrin IB®, Advil®, Nuprin®, and many other brands in 200 mg tablets.

Note: NSAIDs should never be taken together, nor should they be combined with aspirin. NSAIDs have anti-inflammatory effects as well as analgesics. An allergy to aspirin constitutes a contradiction to all the new NSAIDs. Aspirin and the NSAIDs may increase post-treatment bleeding.

Rx

Acetaminophen 325 mg
Disp
Sig: Take 2-3 tablets every 4 hours
Products include: Tylenol®, Datril®, Anacin® 3,
  and many others

Note: Acetaminophen can be given if patient has allergy, bleeding problems, or stomach upset secondary to aspirin or NSAIDs.

Rx

Aleve® 220 mg
Disp
Sig: 1-2 tablets every 8 hours

Ingredient: Naproxen sodium

Rx

Orudis KT® 12.5 mg
Disp
Sig: 1-2 tablets every 8 hours

Ingredient: Ketoprofen

PRESCRIPTION ONLY EXAMPLES

Rx
Motrin® 800 mg*
Disp 16 tablets
Sig: Take 1 tablet 3 times/day

Ingredient: Ibuprofen

Note: For more severe pain, Motrin® (800 mg) can be given up to 4 times/day.

***Note:** Also available as 600 mg

BACTERIAL INFECTIONS

Rx
Penicillin V potassium 500 mg
Disp 28 tablets
Sig: Take 1 tablet 4 times/day

Rx
Amoxicillin 500 mg
Disp 28 tablets
Sig: Take 1 tablet 4 times/day

Rx
Augmentin® 250, 500, or 875 mg
Disp appropriate dose quantity for 7-10 days
Sig: Take 1 tablet 3 times/day for 250 or 500 mg; twice daily for 875 mg

Ingredients: Amoxicillin and clavulanate potassium

Rx
Clarithromycin (Biaxin®) 250 or 500 mg
Disp 14 tablets
Sig: Take 1 tablet every 12 hours until gone

Rx
Zithromax™ (Z-paks) 250 mg
Disp 1 Z-pak (6 capsules)
Sig: 2 capsules first day, then 1 capsule/day for 4 days

Ingredient: Azithromycin

Rx
Cephalexin 250 mg
Disp 28 capsules
Sig: Take 1 capsule 4 times/day

```
Rx

        Dicloxacillin 250 mg
        Disp 28 capsules
        Sig: Take 2 capsules once every 6 hours
```

```
Rx

        Clindamycin 150 mg or 300 mg (Cleocin®)
        Disp 28 capsules
        Sig: Take 1 capsule every 6 hours for orofacial
             infection
```

```
Rx

        Metronidazole 250 mg (Flagyl®)
        Disp 40 tablets
        Sig: Take 1 tablet 4 times/day
```

ANTIMICROBIAL MOUTHRINSES

```
Rx

        Chlorhexidine Gluconate 0.12% (Peridex® and
             PerioGard®)
        Disp 1 bottle
        Sig: 20 mL for 30 seconds 3 times/day
```

```
Rx

        Listerine® (OTC)
        Disp 1 bottle
        Sig: 20 mL for 30 seconds twice daily
```

FUNGAL INFECTIONS

```
Rx

        Mycostatin® oral suspension
        Disp 60 mL (2 oz)
        Sig: Use 1 teaspoonful 4-5 times/day; rinse and
             hold in mouth as long as possible before
             swallowing or spitting out (2 minutes); do not eat
             or drink for 30 minutes following application
```

Ingredient: Nystatin 100,000 units/mL; vehicle contains 50% sucrose and not more than 1% alcohol

---

Rx

Mycostatin® ointment or cream
Disp 15 g or 30 g tube
Sig: Apply liberally to affected areas 4-5 times/day;
    do not eat or drink for 30 minutes after
    application

Note: Denture wearers should apply to dentures prior to each insertion; for edentulous patients, we can also prescribe Mycostatin®
    powder (15 g) to be sprinkled on denture

Ingredients:

Cream: 100,000 units nystatin per g, aqueous vanishing cream base

Ointment: 100,000 units nystatin per g, polyethylene and mineral oil gel base

OR

Rx

Mycelex® troche 10 mg
Disp 70 tablets
Sig: Dissolve 1 tablet in mouth 5 times/day

Ingredient: Clotrimazole

Note: Tablets contain sucrose, risk of caries with prolonged use (>3 months); care must be exercised in diabetic patients

---

Rx

Fungizone® oral suspension
Disp 50 mL
Sig: 1 mL, swish and swallow 4 times/day
    between meals

Ingredient: Amphotericin B

Note: If the patient is refractory to topical treatment, consideration of a systemic route might include Diflucan® or Nizoral®. Also, when
    the patient cannot tolerate topical therapy, ketoconazole (Nizoral®) is an effective, well tolerated, systematic drug for
    mucocutaneous candidiasis. Concern over liver function and possible drug interactions must be considered.

Rx

Nizoral® 200 mg
Disp 10 or 28 tablets
Sig: Take 1 tablet daily for 10-14 days

Ingredient: Ketoconazole

Note: To be used if *Candida* infection does not respond to mycostatin; potential for liver toxicity; liver function should be monitored
    with long-term use (>3 weeks)

Rx

Diflucan® 100 mg
Disp 15 tablets
Sig: Take 2 tablets the first day and 1 tablet daily
    for 10-14 days

Ingredient: Fluconazole

MANAGEMENT OF ANGULAR CHEILITIS

> **Rx**
>
> Nystatin / Triamcinolone (available only as generic)
> Disp 15 g tube
> Sig: Apply to affected area after each meal and
> before bedtime (3-4 times daily)

> **Rx**
>
> Iodoquinol and Hydrocortisone
> Disp 15 g tube
> Sig: Apply locally 3-4 times daily

ORAL VIRAL INFECTIONS

> **Rx**
>
> Acyclovir (Zovirax®) ointment 5% (3%)
> Disp 15 g
> Sig: Apply thin layer to lesions 6 times/day
> for 7 days

Ingredient: Acyclovir

> **Rx**
>
> Acyclovir 200 mg
> Disp 70 capsules
> Sig: Take 1 capsule every 4 hours
> (maximum: 5/day) for 2 weeks

Ingredient: Acyclovir

Note: Use in oral lesions of herpes should be carefully considered by the clinician; see Acyclovir monograph *on page 134*

> **Rx**
>
> Valacyclovir 500 mg tablets
> Disp 8 tablets
> Sig: Take 4 tablets bid (separate doses by 12 hours)
> for recurrent herpes labialis

> **Rx**
>
> Denavir™
> Disp 2 g tube
> Sig: Apply locally every 2 hours during waking hours
> for 4 days

Ingredient: Penciclovir 1%

Note: Denavir™ is recommended for use in herpes labialis

> **Rx**
>
> Abreva™ (OTC) cream
> Sig: Apply locally as directed 5 times/day

Ingredient: 10% docosanol

SUPPORTIVE CARE FOR PAIN AND MAINTENANCE OF NUTRITION DURING ORAL VIRAL INFECTIONS

> **Rx**
>
> Benadryl® elixir 12.5 mg/5 mL
> Disp 4 oz bottle
> Sig: Rinse with 1 teaspoonful for 2 minutes
>   before each meal

Ingredient: Diphenhydramine

> **Rx**
>
> Benadryl® elixir 12.5 mg/5 mL with Kaopectate®,
>   50% mixture by volume
> Disp 8 oz
> Sig: Rinse with 1 teaspoonful every 2 hours

Ingredients: Diphenhydramine and attapulgite

> **Rx**
>
> Xylocaine® viscous 2%
> Disp 450 mL bottle
> Sig: Swish with 1 tablespoon 4 times/day and
>   spit out

Ingredient: Lidocaine

> **Rx**
>
> Meritene®
> Disp 1 lb can (plain, chocolate, eggnog flavors)
> Sig: Take 3 servings daily; prepare as indicated
>   on can

Ingredient: Protein-vitamin-mineral food supplement

BURNING TONGUE SYNDROME, SYMPTOMATIC GEOGRAPHIC TONGUE, MILD-TO-MODERATE FORMS OF ULCERATIONS AND EROSIONS

Burning mouth syndrome is extremely difficult to both diagnose and treat. Initially, systemic factors, including changes in patient's medication, control of diabetes (if the disease is present), concomitant xerostomia, and the presence of fungal infections often complicate the diagnosis and management of burning mouth syndrome. Once these systemic and/or local factors have been eliminated, oftentimes the patient presents with minimal clinically-visible changes and only the subjective complaint of burning mouth. In these instances, a variety of drugs, including clonazepam 0.25-3 mg/day is sometimes used; also the drugs amitriptyline 25-100 mg/day, nortriptyline 10-50 mg/day, gabapentin 900-1500 mg/day, and doxepin as a cream, applied to the lateral borders of the tongue and the areas affected, are sometimes utilized. These drugs should be selected and managed in collaboration with the patient's physician, particularly since many of these patients suffering with burning mouth syndrome have complicated medical histories including the use of additional medications that could be affected.

Elixir of Benadryl®, a potent antihistamine, is used in the oral cavity primarily as a mild topical anesthetic agent for the symptomatic relief of certain allergic deficiencies which should be ruled out as possible etiologies for the oral condition under treatment. It is often used alone as well as in solutions with agents such as Kaopectate® or Maalox® to assist in coating the oral mucosa. Benadryl® can also be used in capsule form.

> **Rx**
>
> Benadryl® elixir 12.5 mg/5 mL
> Disp 4 oz bottle
> Sig: Rinse with 1 teaspoonful for 2 minutes
>   before each meal and swallow

Ingredient: Diphenhydramine

> **Rx**
>
> Benadryl® syrup (mix 50/50) with Kaopectate®*
> Disp 8 oz total
> Sig: Use 2 teaspoons as rinse as needed to
>   relieve pain or burning (use after meals)

*Note: Benadryl can be mixed with Maalox® if constipation is a problem

> **Rx**
>
> Kenalog® in Orabase® 0.1%
> Disp 5 g tube
> Sig: Apply thin layer to affected area 3 times/day

Ingredient: Triamcinolone acetonide

> **Rx**
>
> Lidex® ointment mixed 50/50 with Orabase®
> Disp 30 g total
> Sig: Apply thin layer to oral lesions 4-6 times/day

Ingredient: Fluocinonide 0.05%

Note: To be used for oral inflammatory lesions that do not respond to Kenalog® in Orabase®

> **Rx**
>
> Listerine® antiseptic (OTC)
> 20 mL x 30 sec bid

> **Rx**
>
> Peridex® oral rinse
> Disp 1 bottle
> Sig: 20 mL x 30 sec tid

> **Rx**
>
> PerioGard® oral rinse
> Disp 1 bottle
> Sig: 20 mL x 30 sec tid

> **Rx**
>
> Tetracycline capsules 250 mg
> Disp 40 capsules
> Sig: Suspend contents of 1 capsule in a
> teaspoonful of water; rinse for 2 minutes
> 4 times/day and swallow

Note: Helps to reduce secondary infection of ulcerations

BLISTERING / SLOUGHING LESIONS AND MAJOR ULCERS

Elixir of dexamethasone (Decadron®), a more potent anti-inflammatory agent, is used topically in the management of acute episodes of erosive lichen planus and major aphthae. Continued supervision of the patient during treatment is essential.

> **Rx**
>
> Decadron® elixir 0.5 mg/5 mL
> Disp 100 mL bottle
> Sig: Rinse with 1 teaspoonful for 2 minutes
> 4 times/day; do not swallow

Ingredient: Dexamethasone

Other regimens altering topical and systemic uptake can be designed by the dentist depending upon the severity and usual duration of the lesions

Systemic steroids may be considered:

> **Rx**
>
> Prednisone 5 mg
> Disp 60 tablets
> Sig: Take 4 tablets in morning and 4 tablets at
> noon for 4 days; then decrease the total number
> of tablets by 1 each day until down to zero

Caution: Take medication with food

Note: Medrol® (methylprednisolone) dose packs (2-60 mg/day) is an alternative choice; see Methylprednisolone monograph *on page 143*

For a high-potency, topical corticosteroid:

> **Rx**
>
> Temovate® cream 0.05%
> Disp 15 g tube
> Sig: Apply locally 4-6 times/day

Ingredient: Clobetasol

ANTICARIES AGENTS

Toothpastes with triclosan such as Colgate Total® show promise for combined treatment/prevention of caries, plaque, and gingivitis.

FLUORIDE GELS

Used for the prevention of demineralization of the tooth structure secondary to xerostomia. For patients with long-term or permanent xerostomia, daily application is accomplished using custom gel applicator trays. Patients with porcelain crowns should use a neutral pH fluoride (see Fluoride Preparations *on page 161*).

SPECIAL TOPICS

Management of Patients Undergoing Cancer Therapy 156

Dry Mouth (Xerostomia) 159

Fluorides 161

Preprocedural Antibiotics in Dental Patients 162

HIV Infection and AIDS...166

Normal Blood Values 167

Suggested Readings 168

MANAGEMENT OF PATIENTS UNDERGOING CANCER THERAPY
AND THOSE WITH CHRONIC DRY MOUTH OR XEROSTOMIA

CANCER PATIENT DENTAL PROTOCOL

The objective in the treatment of a patient with cancer is the eradication of the disease. Oral complications, such as mucosal ulceration, xerostomia, bleeding, and infections can cause significant morbidity and may compromise the systemic treatment of the patient. With proper oral evaluation before systemic treatment, many of the complications can be minimized or prevented.

MUCOSITIS

Normal oral mucosa acts as a barrier against chemical and food irritants and against oral microorganisms. The disruption of the mucosal barrier can, therefore, lead to secondary infection, increased pain, delayed healing, and decreased nutritional intake.

Mucositis is inflammation of the mucous membranes. It is a common reaction to chemotherapy and radiation therapy. It is first seen as an erythematous patch. The mucosal epithelium becomes thin as a result of the killing of the rapidly dividing basal layer mucosal cells. Seven to 10 days after cytoreduction chemotherapy and between 1000 cGy and 3000 cGy of radiation to the head and neck, mucosal tissues begin to desquamate and eventually develop into frank ulcerations. The mucosal integrity is broken and then is secondarily infected by the normal oral flora. The resultant ulcerations can also act as a portal of entry for pathogenic organisms into the patient's bloodstream and may lead to systemic infections. These ulcerations often force interruption of therapy.

Certain chemotherapeutic agents, such as 5-fluorouracil, methotrexate, and doxorubicin are more commonly associated with the development of oral mucositis. Treatment of oral mucositis is mainly palliative, but steps should be taken to minimize secondary pathogenic infections. Culture and sensitivity data should be obtained to select the appropriate therapy for the bacterial, viral, or fungal organisms found.

Prevention of radiation mucositis is difficult. Stents can be constructed to prevent the irradiation of uninvolved tissues. The use of multiple ports and fractionation of the therapy into smaller doses over a longer period of time can reduce the severity. Fractured restorations, sharp teeth, and ill-fitted prostheses can damage the soft tissues and lead to additional interruption of mucosal barriers. Correction of these problems before radiation therapy can diminish these complications.

CHEMOTHERAPY

Chemotherapy for neoplasia also frequently results in oral complications. Infections and mucositis are the most common complications seen in patients receiving chemotherapy. Also occurring frequently are pain, altered nutrition, and xerostomia, which can significantly affect the quality of life of the patient.

RADIATION CARIES

Dental caries that sometimes follows radiation therapy is called radiation caries. It usually develops in the cervical region of the teeth adjacent to the gingiva. It often affects many teeth. It is secondary to the damage done to the salivary glands and is initiated by dental plaque, but its rapid progress is due to changes in saliva. In addition to the diminution in the amount of saliva, both the salivary pH and buffering capacity are diminished, which decreases the anticaries activity of saliva. Oral bacteria also changes with xerostomia, leading to the increase in caries activity.

SALIVARY CHANGES

Chemotherapy is not thought to directly alter salivary flow, but alterations in taste and subjective sensations of dry mouth are relatively common complaints. Patients with mucositis and those with graft-vs-host disease following bone marrow or stem cell transplantation often demonstrate signs and symptoms of xerostomia. Radiation does directly affect salivary production. Radiation to the salivary glands produces fibrosis and alters the production of saliva. If all the major salivary glands are in the field, the decrease in saliva can be dramatic and the serous portion of the glands seems to be most severely affected. The saliva produced is increased in viscosity, which contributes to food retention and increased plaque formation. These xerostomic patients have difficulty in managing a normal diet. Normal saliva also has bacteriostatic properties that are diminished in these patients.

The dental management recommendations for patients undergoing chemotherapy, bone marrow transplantation, and/or radiation therapy for the treatment of cancer are based primarily on clinical observations. The following protocols will provide a conservative, consistent approach to the dental management of patients undergoing chemotherapy or bone marrow transplantation. Many of the cancer chemotherapy drugs produce oral side effects including mucositis, oral ulceration, dry mouth, acute infections, and taste aberrations. Cancer drugs include antibiotics, alkylating agents, antimetabolites, DNA inhibitors, hormones, and cytokines.

All patients undergoing chemotherapy or bone marrow transplantation for malignant disease should have the following baseline:

A. Panoramic radiograph

B. Dental consultation and examination

C. Dental prophylaxis and cleaning (if the neutrophil count is >1500/mm^3 and the platelet count is >50,000/mm^3)

- Prophylaxis and cleaning will be deferred if the patient's neutrophil count is <1500 and the platelet count is <50,000. Oral hygiene recommendations will be made. These levels are arbitrary guidelines and the dentist should consider the patient's oral condition and planned procedure relative to hemorrhage and level of bacteremia.

D. Oral Hygiene. Patients should be encouraged to follow normal hygiene procedures. Addition of a chlorhexidine mouth rinse such as Peridex® or PerioGard® *on page 138* is usually helpful. If the patient develops oral mucositis, tolerance of such alcohol-based products may be limited.

E. If the patient develops mucositis, bacterial, viral, and fungal cultures should be obtained. Sucralfate suspension in either a pharmacy prepared form or Carafate® suspension as well as Benadryl® *on page 140* or Xylocaine® viscous *on page 143* can assist in helping the patient to tolerate food. Patients may also require systemic analgesics for pain relief depending on the presence of mucositis. Positive fungal cultures may require a nystatin swish and swallow prescription.

F. The determination of performing dental procedures must be based on the goal of preventing infection during periods of neutropenia. Timing of procedures must be coordinated with the patient's hematologic status.

G. If oral surgery is required, at least 7-10 days of healing should be allowed before the anticipated date of bone marrow suppression (eg, ANC <1000/mm^3 and/or platelet count of 50,000/mm^3).

H. Daily use of topical fluorides is recommended for those who have received radiation therapy to the head-neck region involving salivary glands. Any patients with prolonged xerostomia subsequent to graft-vs-host disease and/or chemotherapy can also be considered for fluoride supplement. Use the fluoride-containing mouthwashes (Act®, Fluorigard®, etc - see Fluorides in this section) each night before going to sleep; swish, hold 1-2 minutes, spit out or use prescription fluorides (gels or rinses); apply them daily for 3-4 minutes as directed; if the mouth is sore (mucositis), use flavorless/colorless gels (Thera-Flur®, Gel-Kam®). Improvement in salivary flow following radiation therapy to the head and neck has been noted with Salagen® *on page 145* or Evoxac™ *on page 137*.

ORAL LESIONS IN CANCER TREATMENT

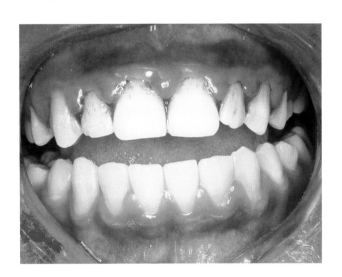

Oral hemorrhage, resulting from a platelet deficiency, in a patient receiving myelosuppressive chemotherapy for the treatment of leukemia

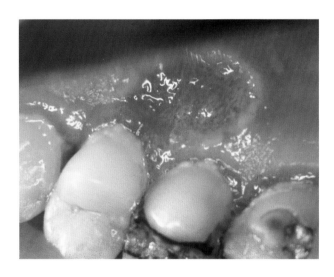

Oral mucositis, resulting from reactivation of herpes simplex virus, in a patient receiving myelosuppressive chemotherapy in preparation for bone marrow transplantation

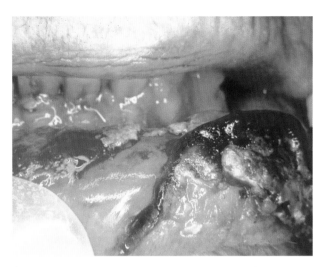

Oral mucositis, resulting from mucosal thinning and ulcerations complicated by fungal overgrowth, in a patient receiving myelosuppressive chemotherapy in preparation for bone marrow transplantation

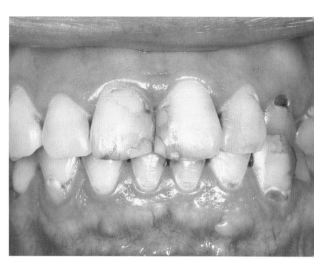

Chronic xerostomia, subsequent to ionizing radiation, in a patient being treated for laryngeal cancer, resulting in high caries activity

DRY MOUTH (XEROSTOMIA)

Fungal colonization and systemic considerations (eg, Sjögren's disease) also play a role in successful management. Dry mouth associated with radiation therapy, drug therapy, aging, and Sjögren's disease may be managed by rinsing with a solution of sodium carboxymethylcellulose. It is a nonirritating agent that moistens and lubricates the oral tissues and may be used for prolonged periods of time without adverse effects. For dentulous patients, fluoride and electrolytes have been added to this solution to reduce caries susceptibility (Xero-Lube®). Consideration of alternative medical drug regimens in consult with the physician may assist in management. Numerous patients being treated for anxiety or depression are often susceptible to chronic xerostomia due to medications selected.

ARTIFICIAL SALIVA PRODUCTS

Common US Brand Name Glandosane® Mouth Moisturizer
Manufacturer Kenwood Laboratories
Product Type Aqueous solution sprayed into the mouth
Manufacturer's Description Mouth moisturizer to relieve dry mouth or throat associated with various conditions; available as unflavored, lemon, or mint
Indication Hyposalivation, xerostomia; relieves dry mouth and throat
Ingredients Water, sodium carboxymethylcellulose (0.500 g), sorbitol (1.500 g), sodium chloride (0.042 g), potassium chloride (0.060 g), calcium chloride dihydrate (0.007 g), magnesium chloride hexahydrate (0.003 g), dipotassium hydrogen phosphate (0.017 g)
Directions for Use Spray directly into mouth or throat for 1-2 seconds; use as needed
Supply and Purchase 50 mL cans of aqueous solution; available at pharmacies or through manufacturer

Common US Brand Name Moi-Stir® Moistening Solution
Manufacturer Kingswood Laboratories, Inc
Product Type Pump spray
Manufacturer's Description Saliva supplement in a 4 oz pump spray bottle for lubrication and moistening of the mouth and mucosal area
Indication Nontherapeutic treatment of dry mouth, intended for comfort only
Ingredients Water, sorbitol, sodium carboxymethylcellulose, methylparaben, propylparaben, potassium chloride, sodium chloride, and flavor
Directions for Use Spray directly into mouth as necessary to treat drying conditions
Supply and Purchase 4 oz spray bottle; order directly from Kingswood Laboratories, Inc or from various distributors

Common US Brand Name MouthKote® Oral Moisturizer
Manufacturer Parnell Pharmaceuticals, Inc
Product Type Aqueous solution
Manufacturer's Description Oral moisturizer for dry mouth conditions caused by medications, disease, surgery, irradiation or aging
Indication Treating discomfort of oral dryness
Ingredients Water, xylitol, sorbitol, yerba santa, citric acid, ascorbic acid, flavor, sodium benzoate, sodium saccharin
Directions for Use Swirl 1 or 2 teaspoonfuls in mouth for 8-10 seconds, then swallow or spit out; shake well before using
Supply and Purchase 2 oz. and 8 oz bottles; order from manufacturer

Common US Brand Name Nighttime Spray®
Manufacturer Omnii International
Product Type Spray bottle
Manufacturer's Description Plaque fighting spray for use at night
Indication Treating the discomfort of oral dryness
Directions for Use Spray in mouth before retiring; spread over teeth and tissue with tongue
Supply and Purchase 35 mL spray bottle; order direct from the manufacturer

Common US Brand Name Optimoist™ Oral Moisturizer
Manufacturer Colgate Oral Pharmaceuticals
Product Type Oral moisturizer, aqueous solution
Manufacturer's Description Pleasant tasting saliva substitute that provides instant relief for dry mouth and dry throat sufferers
Indication Treating the discomfort of oral dryness without demineralizing tooth enamel
Ingredients Deionized water, xylitol, calcium phosphate monobasic, citric acid, sodium hydroxide, sodium benzoate, flavor, acesulfame potassium, hydroxyethylcellulose, polysorbate 20 and sodium monofluorophosphate. Fluoride concentration is 2 parts per million
Directions for Use Spray into mouth to relieve dry mouth discomfort as needed; may be swallowed or expectorated
Supply and Purchase 2 and 12 oz bottles; mass merchandise stores, food stores and drugstores

Common US Brand Name Biotene® OralBalance" Mouth Moisturizing Gel
Manufacturer Laclede Professional Products, Inc
Product Type Gel
Manufacturer's Description Oral lubricant specially formulated to help promote healing as it moistens; contains the "Biotene" protective salivary enzyme system; relieves dry mouth up to 8 hours; coats sore, inflamed tissues to promote healing; helps speech and swallowing
Indication Treat symptoms of dry mouth; for relief of symptoms of dry mouth burning, sore tissue palate and swallowing difficulties
Ingredients Glucose oxidase (2000 units), lactoperoxidase (3000 units), lysozyme (5 mg), lactoferrin (5 mg); Other: Hydrogenated starch, xylitol, hydroxyethyl cellulose, glycerate polyhydrate, aloe vera
Directions for Use Use whenever necessary to relieve dryness; using a clean fingertip, apply a one inch ribbon of gel onto tongue, and add additional amount of gel on affected areas
Supply and Purchase 1.4 oz tube; available from mass merchandise stores, food stores and drugstores

Common US Brand Name Salivart® Synthetic Saliva, Aqueous Solution
Manufacturer Gebauer Co
Product Type Aerosol aqueous spray
Manufacturer's Description Oral moisturizer used as replacement therapy for patients complaining of xerostomia no matter what the cause
Indication Replacement therapy for patients with reduced salivary flow
Ingredients Sodium carboxymethylcellulose, sorbitol, sodium chloride, potassium chloride, calcium chloride dihydrate, magnesium chloride hexahydrate, potassium phosphate dibasic, purified water, propellant: nitrogen
Directions for Use Spray directly into mouth or throat for 1-2 seconds; use as often as needed to maintain moistness
Supply and Purchase 2.48 fl oz (75 g); available from most pharmacies or from manufacturer

OTHER DRY MOUTH PRODUCTS

Common US Brand Name Biotene® Dry Mouth Gum
Manufacturer Laclede Professional Products, Inc
Product Type Chewing gum
Manufacturer's Description When used daily, the active enzymes in Biotene can be effective in helping the defense system normally found in saliva
Indication Use to treat oral dryness
Ingredients Lactoperoxidase (0.11 units), glucose oxidase (0.15 units); Other: Sorbitol, gum base, xylitol, hydrogenated glucose, potassium thiocyanate
Directions for Use Chew one or two pieces, as required, to relieve dry mouth or throat
Supply and Purchase Each package contains 17 pieces; available from pharmacies or from manufacturer

Common US Brand Name Biotene® Dry Mouth Toothpaste

Manufacturer Laclede Professional products, Inc

Product Type Toothpaste

Manufacturer's Description To be used in place of your regular toothpaste to reduce harmful bacteria, to boost and replenish defense systems normally found in saliva

Indication To be used in place of your regular toothpaste for cleansing action

Ingredients Lactoperoxidase (15,000 units), glucose oxidase (10,000 units), lysozyme (16 mg), sodium monofluorophosphate; Other: Sorbitol, glycerin, calcium pyrophosphate, hydrated silica, xylitol, isoceteth-20, cellulose gum, flavor, sodium benzoate, beta-d-glucose, potassium thiocyanate

Directions for Use Use in place of regular toothpaste on a daily basis, especially at night

Supply and Purchase 4.5 oz tube; available from pharmacies or from manufacturer

Common US Brand Name Biotene® Gentle Mouthwash

Manufacturer Laclede Professional products, Inc

Product Type Mouthwash

Manufacturer's Description Mouthwash especially beneficial to individuals experiencing dry mouth or having oral irritations

Indication Mouthwash for treatment of dry mouth or oral irritations

Ingredients Lysozyme, lactoferrin, glucose oxidase, lactoperoxidase

Directions for Use Use 15 mL (one tablespoonful); swish thoroughly for 30 seconds and spit out. If throat is dry, sip one tablespoonful of mouthwash 2-3 times daily.

Supply and Purchase Available from pharmacies or from manufacturer

Common US Brand Name Moi-Stir® Oral Swabsticks

Manufacturer Kingswood Laboratories, Inc

Product Type Premoistened swabsticks

Manufacturer's Description Premoistened swabsticks for lubrication and moistening of the mouth and mucosal area

Indication Nontherapeutic treatment of dry mouth, intended for comfort only

Ingredients Water, sorbitol, sodium carboxymethylcellulose, methylparaben, propylparaben, potassium chloride, sodium chloride and flavor

Directions for Use Gently swab all intraoral surfaces of mouth, gums, tongue, palate, buccal mucosa, gingival, teeth, and lips when uncomfortably drying conditions exist

Supply and Purchase 3 swabsticks per packet, 100 packets per case; order directly from Kingswood Laboratories, Inc. or from various distributors

CHOLINERGIC SALIVARY STIMULANTS (Rx only)

Pilocarpine (Salagen®) is indicated for the treatment of xerostomia caused by radiation therapy in patients with head and neck cancer and for the treatment of xerostomia in patients suffering from Sjögren's syndrome. The usual dosage in adults is 5 mg tablets, 1-2 tablets 3-4 times daily not to exceed 30 mg/day. **Note:** Patients should be treated for a minimum of 90 days to achieve clinical effects.

Cevimeline (Evoxac™) is indicated for the treatment of symptoms of dry mouth in patients with Sjögren's syndrome. The usual dosage in adults is 30 mg 3 times daily. Cevimeline (Evoxac™) is supplied in 30 mg capsules.

FLUORIDES

Common US Brand Names ACT® (OTC); Duraflor® Cavity Varnish; Fluor-A-Day®; Fluorigard® (OTC); Fluorinse®; Fluoritab®; Flura-Drops®; Flura-Loz®; Gel-Kan®; Gel-Tin® (OTC); Karidium®; Karigel®; Karigel®-N; Listermint® with Fluoride (OTC); Luride®; Luride® Lozi-Tab®; Luride®-SF Lozi-Tab®; Minute-Gel®; Pediaflor®; Pharmaflur®; Phos-Flur®; Point-Two®; PreviDent®; Stop® (OTC); Thera-Flur®; Thera-Flur-N®

Canadian Brand Names Fluor-A-Day®; Fluotic®; Pedi-Dent™;
Indication Prevention of dental caries
Dosage Forms Fluoride ion content is listed in brackets

PRESCRIPTION ONLY (Rx) PRODUCTS

Form	Brand Name	Strength / Size
Drops, oral (as sodium)		0.275 mg/drop [0.125 mg/drop]
	Fluoritab®, Flura-Drops®	0.55 mg/drop [0.25 mg/drop] (22.8 mL, 24 mL)
	Karidium®, Luride®	0.275 mg/drop [0.125 mg/drop] (30 mL, 60 mL)
	Pediaflor®	1.1 mg/mL [0.5 mg/mL] (50 mL)
Gel-Drops	Thera-Flur® (lime-flavored), Thera-Flur-N®	1.1% [0.55%] (24 mL)
Gel, topical		
Acidulated phosphate fluoride	Minute-Gel® (spearmint, strawberry, grape, apple-cinnamon, cherry cola, bubblegum flavors)	1.23% (480 mL)
Sodium fluoride	Karigel® (orange flavor)	1.1% [0.5%]
	Karigel®-N	1.1% [0.5%]
	PreviDent® (mint, berry, cherry, fruit sherbet flavors)	1.1% [0.5%] (24 g, 30 g, 60 g, 120 g, 130 g, 250 g)
Lozenge (as sodium)	Flura-Loz® (raspberry flavor)	2.2 mg [1 mg]
Rinse, topical (as sodium)	Fluorinse®, Point-Two®	0.2% [0.09%] (240 mL, 480 mL, 3780 mL)
Solution, oral (as sodium)	Phos-Flur® (cherry, cinnamon, grape, wintergreen flavors)	0.44 mg/mL [0.2 mg/mL] (250 mL, 500 mL, 3780 mL)
Tablet (as sodium)		1.1 mg [0.5 mg]; 2.2 mg [1 mg]
	Fluor-A-Day®	0.55 mg [0.25 mg]
Chewable	Fluor-A-Day®, Fluoritab®, Luride® Lozi-Tab®, Pharmaflur®	1.1 mg [0.5 mg]
	Fluor-A-Day®, Fluoritab®, Karidium®, Luride® Lozi-Tab®, Luride®-SF Lozi-Tab®, Pharmaflur®	2.2 mg [1 mg]
Oral	Flura®, Karidium®	2.2 mg [1 mg]
Varnish	Duraflor®	5% [50 mg/mL] (10 mL)

OVER-THE-COUNTER (OTC) PRODUCTS

Form	Brand Name	Strength / Size
Gel, topical (stannous fluoride)	Gel-Kam® (cinnamon, fruit, mint flavors)	0.4% [0.1%] (65 g, 105 gm 122 g)
	Gel-Tin® (lime, grape, cinnamon, raspberry, mint, orange flavors)	0.4% [0.1%] (60 g, 120 g)
	Stop® (grape, cinnamon, bubblegum, pina colada, mint flavors)	0.4% [0.1%] (60 g, 120 g)
Rinse, topical (as sodium)	ACT®, Fluorigard®	0.05% [0.02%] (90 mL, 180 mL, 300 mL, 360 mL, 480 mL)
	Listermint® with Fluoride	0.02% [0.01%] (180 mL, 300 mL, 360 mL, 480 mL, 540 mL, 720 mL, 960 mL, 1740 mL)

PREPROCEDURAL ANTIBIOTICS IN DENTAL PATIENTS

In dental practice the clinician is often confronted with a decision to prescribe antibiotics. The focus of this chapter is on the use of antibiotics as a preprocedural treatment in the prevention of adverse infectious sequelae in the two most commonly encountered situations: prevention of endocarditis and prosthetic implants.

The criteria for preprocedural decisions begins with patient evaluation. An accurate and complete medical history is always the initial basis for any prescriptive treatments on the part of the dentist. These prescriptive treatments can include ordering appropriate laboratory tests, referral to the patient's physician for consultation, or immediate decision to prescribe preprocedural antibiotics. The dentist should also be aware that antibiotic coverage of the patient might be appropriate due to diseases that are covered elsewhere

in this text, such as human immunodeficiency virus cavernous thrombosis, undiagnosed or uncontrolled diabetes, lupus, renal failure, and periods of neutropenia a are often associated with cancer chemotherapy. In these instances, medical consultation is almost always necessary in making antibiotic decisions in order to tailor the treatment and dosing to the individual patient's needs.

All tables or figures in this chapter were adapted from the ADA Advisory Statement: "Antibiotic Prophylaxis for Dental Patients With Total Joint Replacement," *J Am Dent Assoc* 1997, 128:1004-8 or from Dajani AS, Taubert KA, Wilson W, et al, "Prevention of Bacterial Endocarditis. Recommendations by the American Heart Association," *JAMA*, 1997 7(22):1794-801.

Table 1.
DENTAL PROCEDURES AND PREPROCEDURAL ANTIBIOTICS

Endocarditis or Prosthesis Prophylaxis Recommended Due to Likely Significant Bacteremia*
Dental extractions
Periodontal procedures including surgery, subgingival placement of antibiotic fibers/strips, scaling and root planing, probing, recall maintenance
Dental implant placement and reimplantation of avulsed teeth
Endodontic (root canal) instrumentation or surgery only beyond the apex
Initial placement of orthodontic bands but not brackets
Intraligamentary local anesthetic injections
Prophylactic cleaning of teeth or implants where bleeding is anticipated
Endocarditis Prophylaxis Not Recommended Due to Usually Insignificant Bacteremia
Restorative dentistry† (operative and prosthodontic) with or without retraction cord‡
Local anesthetic injections (nonintraligamentary)
Intracanal endodontic treatment; postplacement and build-up‡
Placement of rubber dam‡
Postoperative suture removal
Placement of removable prosthodontic/orthodontic appliances
Oral impressions‡
Fluoride treatments
Taking of oral radiographs
Orthodontic appliance adjustment
Shedding of primary teeth
‡In general, the presence of moderate to severe gingival inflammation may elevate these procedures to a higher risk of bacteremia.

*Prophylaxis is recommended for patients with high- and moderate-risk cardiac as well as high-risk prosthesis conditions

†This includes restoration of decayed teeth and replacement of missing teeth

‡Clinical judgment may indicate antibiotic use in any circumstances that may create significant bleeding.

Table 2.
CARDIAC CONDITIONS PREDISPOSING TO ENDOCARDITIS

Endocarditis Prophylaxis Recommended
High-Risk Category
Prosthetic cardiac valves, including bioprosthetic and homograft valves
Previous bacterial endocarditis
Complex cyanotic congenital heart disease (eg, single ventricle states, transposition of the great arteries, tetralogy of Fallot)
Surgically constructed systemic pulmonary shunts or conduits
Moderate-Risk Category
Most other congenital cardiac malformations (other than above and below)
Acquired valvar dysfunction (eg, rheumatic heart disease)
Hypertrophic cardiomyopathy
Mitral valve prolapse with valvar regurgitation and/or thickened leaflets*
Endocarditis Prophylaxis Not Recommended
Negligible-Risk Category (no greater risk than the general population)
Isolated secundum atrial septal defect
Surgical repair of atrial septal defect, ventricular septal defect, or patent ductus arteriosus (without residual defects beyond 6 mo)
Previous coronary artery bypass graft surgery
Mitral valve prolapse without valvar regurgitation
Physiologic, functional, or innocent heart murmurs
Previous Kawasaki disease without valvar dysfunction
Previous rheumatic fever without valvar dysfunction
Cardiac pacemakers (intravascular and epicardial) and implanted defibrillators
**Specific risk for patients with a history of fenfluramine or dexfenfluramine (fen-phen or Redux®) use, has not been determined. Such patients should have medical evaluation for potential cardiac damage, as currently recommended by the FDA.

Table 3.
PATIENTS WITH POTENTIAL ELEVATED RISK OF JOINT INFECTION

Inflammatory arthropathies: Rheumatoid arthritis, systemic lupus erythematosus
Disease-, drug-, or radiation-induced immunosuppression
Insulin-dependent diabetes
First 2 years following joint replacement
Previous prosthetic joint infections
Patients with acute infections at a distant site
Hemophilia
Malnourishment*
Patients with malignancies*
Patients with HIV infection*

*Source: American Dental Association; American Academy of Orthopedic Surgeons, "Antibiotic Prophylaxis for Dental Patients With Total Joint Replacements," *J Am Dent Assoc*, 2003, 134(7):895-9.

Figure 1
Preprocedural Dental Action Plan for Patients With a History
Indicative of Elevated Endocarditis Risk

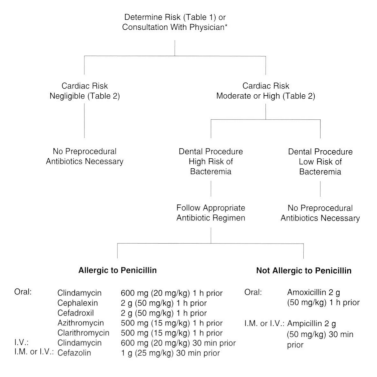

Dosages for children are in parentheses and should never exceed adult dose. Cephalosporins should be avoided in patients with previous Type I hypersensitivity reactions to penicillin due to some evidence of cross allergenicity.

* For Emergency Dental Care, the clinician should attempt phone consultation. If unable to contact patient's physician or determine risk, the patient should be treated as though there is moderate or high risk of cardiac complication and follow the algorithm.

Figure 2
Patient With Suspected Mitral Valve Prolapse

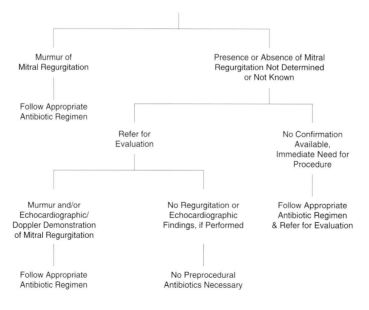

Figure 3
Preprocedural Dental Action Plan for
Patients With Prosthetic Implants

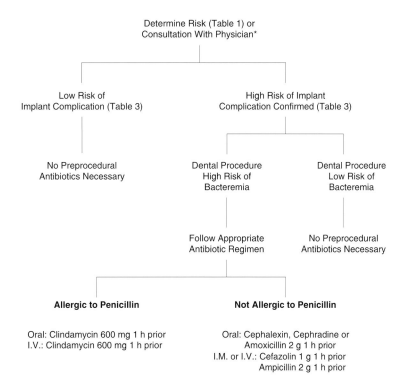

Cephalosporins should be avoided in patients with previous Type I hypersensitivity reactions to penicillin due to some evidence of cross allergenicity.

*For Emergency Dental Care the clinician should attempt phone consultation. If unable to contact patient's physician or determine risk, the patient should be treated as though there is high risk of implant complication and follow the algorithm.

HIV INFECTION AND AIDS

NATURAL HISTORY OF HIV INFECTION/ORAL MANIFESTATIONS

Time From Transmission (Average)	Observation	CD4 Cell Count
0	Viral transmissions	Normal: 1000 ($\pm$500/mm^3)
2-4 weeks	Self-limited infectious mononucleosis-like illness with fever, rash, leukopenia, mucocutaneous ulcerations (mouth, genitals, etc), thrush	Transient decrease
6-12 weeks	Seroconversion (rarely requires $\geq$3 months for seroconversion)	Normal
0-8 years	Healthy/asymptomatic HIV infection; peripheral/persistent generalized lymphadenopathy; HPV, thrush, OHL; RAU, periodontal diseases, salivary gland diseases; dermatitis	$\geq$500/mm^3 gradual reduction with average decrease of 50-80/mm^3/year
4-8 years	Early symptomatic HIV infection previously called (AIDS-related complex): Thrush, vaginal candidiasis (persistent, frequent and/or severe), cervical dysplasia/CA Hodgkin's lymphoma, B-cell lymphoma, oral hairy leukoplakia, salivary gland diseases, ITP, xerostomia, dermatitis, shingles; RAU, herpes simplex, HPV, bacterial infections, periodontal diseases, molluscum contagiosum, other physical symptoms: fever, weight loss, fatigue	$\geq$300-500/mm^3
6-10 years	AIDS: Wasting syndrome, *Candida* esophagitis, Kaposi's sarcoma, HIV-associated dementia, disseminated *M. avium*, Hodgkin's or B-cell lymphoma, herpes simplex >30 days; PCP; cryptococcal meningitis, other systemic fungal infections; CMV	<200/mm^3

Natural history indicates course of HIV infection in absence of antiretroviral treatment. Adapted from Bartlett JG, "A Guide to HIV Care from the AIDS Care Program of the Johns Hopkins Medical Institutions," 2001.

PCP - *Pneumocystis carinii* pneumonia; ITP - idiopathic thrombocytopenia purpura; HPV - human papilloma virus; OHL - oral hairy leukoplakia; RAU - recurrent aphthous ulcer

CD4+ LYMPHOCYTE COUNT AND PERCENTAGE AS RELATED TO THE RISK OF OPPORTUNISTIC INFECTION

CD4+ Cells/mm^3	CD4+ Percentage*	Risk of Opportunistic Infection
>600	32-60	No increased risk
400-500	<29	Initial immune suppression
200-400	14-28	Appearance of opportunistic infections, some may be major
<200	<14	Severe immune suppression. AIDS diagnosis. Major opportunistic infections. Although variable, prognosis for surviving more than 3 years is poor.
<50	—	Although variable, prognosis for surviving more than 1 year is poor

*Several studies have suggested that the CD4+ percentage demonstrates less variability between measurements, as compared to the absolute CD4+ cell count. CD4+ percentages may therefore give a clearer impression of the course of disease.

Adapted from Glick M and Silverman S, "Dental Management of HIV-Infected Patients," *J Am Dent Assoc* (Supplement to Reviewers), 1995.

ORAL LESIONS COMMONLY SEEN IN HIV/AIDS

Condition
Oral candidiasis
Angular cheilitis
Oral hairy leukoplakia
Periodontal diseases
Linear gingivitis
Ulcerative periodontitis
Herpes simplex
Herpes zoster
Chronic aphthous ulceration
Salivary gland disease
Human papillomavirus
Kaposi's sarcoma
Non-Hodgkin's lymphoma
Tuberculosis

NORMAL BLOOD VALUES

Test	Range of Normal Values
Complete blood count (CBC)	
White blood cells	4,500-11,000
Red blood cells (male)	$4.6\text{-}6.2 \times 10^6$ μL
Red blood cells (female)	$4.2\text{-}5.4 \times 10^6$ μL
Platelets	150,000-450,000
Hematocrit (male)	40% to 54%
Hematocrit (female)	38% to 47%
Hemoglobin (male)	13.5-18 g/dL
Hemoglobin (female)	12-16 g/dL
Mean corpuscular volume (MCV)	80-96 μm^3
Mean corpuscular hemoglobin (MCH)	27-31 pg
Mean corpuscular hemoglobin concentration (MCHC)	32% to 36%
Differential white blood cell count (%)	
Segmented neutrophils	56
Bands	3.0
Eosinophils	2.7
Basophils	0.3
Lymphocytes	34.0
Monocytes	4.0
Hemostasis	
Bleeding time (BT)	2-8 minutes
Prothrombin time (PT)	10-13 seconds
Activated partial thromboplastin time (aPTT)	25-35 seconds
Serum chemistry	
Glucose (fasting)	70-110 mg/dL
Blood urea nitrogen (BUN)	8-23 mg/dL
Creatinine (male)	0.1-0.4 mg/dL
Creatinine (female)	0.2-0.7 mg/dL
Bilirubin, indirect (unconjugated)	0.3 mg/dL
Bilirubin, direct (conjugated)	0.1-1 mg/dL
Calcium	9.2-11 mg/dL
Magnesium	1.8-3 mg/dL
Phosphorus	2.3-4.7 mg/dL
Serum electrolytes	
Sodium (Na^+)	136-142 mEq/L
Potassium (K^+)	3.8-5 mEq/L
Chloride (Cl^-)	95-103 mEq/L
Bicarbonate (HCO_3^-)	21-28 mmol/L
Serum enzymes	
Alkaline phosphatase	20-130 IU/L
Alanine aminotransferase (ALT) (formerly called SGPT)	4-36 units/L
Aspartate aminotransferase (AST) (formerly called SGOT)	8-33 units/L
Amylase	16-120 Somogyi units/dL
Creatine kinase (CK) (male)	55-170 units/L
Creatine kinase (CK) (female)	30-135 units/L

SUGGESTED READINGS

TEXTBOOKS

ADA Guide to Dental Therapeutics, 2nd ed, Chicago, IL: ADA Publishing, 2000.

Bartlett JG and Gallant JE, *Medical Management of HIV Infection*, Baltimore, MD: Johns Hopkins University, 2000.

Boyd RF, *Basic Medical Microbiology*, 5th ed, Boston, MA: Little, Brown and Company, 1995.

Cawson RA and Eveson J, *Oral Pathology and Diagnosis: Color Atlas with Integrated Text*, Philadelphia, PA: WB Saunders Co, 1987.

Clinician's Guide to Treatment of Common Oral Conditions, 4th ed, Rosenberg SW and Arm RN (eds), New York, NY: The American Academy of Oral Medicine, 1997.

Clinician's Guide to Treatment of Medically-Compromised Dental Patients, Tyler MT and Lozada-Nur F (eds), New York, NY: The American Academy of Oral Medicine, 1995.

Eisen D and Lynch DP, *The Mouth: Diagnosis and Treatment*, St Louis, MO: Mosby, Inc, 1998.

Eversole LR, *Oral Medicine: A Pocket Guide*, Philadelphia, PA: WB Saunders Co, 1996.

Handbook of Supportive Care in Cancer, 2nd ed, Klastersky J, Schimpff SC, and Senn HJ (eds), New York, NY: Marcel Dekker, Inc, 1999.

Little JW, Palace DA, Miller CS, et al, *Dental Management of the Medically Compromised Patient*, 5th ed, St Louis, MO: Mosby, Inc, 1997.

Neville BW, Damm DD, Allen CM, et al, *Oral & Maxillofacial Pathology*, Philadelphia, PA: WB Saunders Co, 1995.

Newland JR, "Diseases of the Mouth," *Conn's Current Therapy 2000*, Rakel RE and Bope ET (eds), Philadelphia, PA: WB Saunders Co, 2000.

Principles and Practice of Infectious Diseases, 5th ed, Mandell GL, Bennett JE, and Dolin R (eds), New York, NY: Churchill Livingstone, 2000.

Regezi JA and Sciubba JJ, *Oral Pathology: Clinical Pathologic Correlations*, 3rd ed, Philadelphia, PA: WB Saunders Co, 1999.

Silverman S, Jr, *Color Atlas of Oral Manifestations of AIDS*, 2nd ed, Toronto, Canada: BC Decker, Inc, 1996.

Tyldesley WR, *Color Atlas of Oral Medicine*, 2nd ed, Barcelona, Spain: Mosby-Wolfe Publishing, 1994.

Wood NK, *Review of Diagnosis, Oral Medicine, Radiology, and Treatment Planning*, 4th ed, St Louis, MO: Mosby, Inc, 1999.

Wray D and Gibson J, *Colour Guide, Picture Tests: Oral Medicine*, Edinburgh, UK: Churchill Livingstone, 1997.

Wray D, Lowe GD, Dagg JH, et al, *Textbook of General and Oral Medicine*, Edinburgh, UK: Churchill Livingstone, 1999.

Wynn RL, Meiller TF, and Crossley HL, *Drug Information Handbook for Dentistry*, 6th ed, Hudson, OH: Lexi-Comp, Inc, 2000.

BLISTERING / SLOUGHING LESIONS

Allen CM and Camisa C, "Paraneoplastic Pemphigus: A Review of the Literature," *Oral Dis*, 2000, 6(4):208-14 (review).

Anhalt GJ, "Pemphigoid: Bullous and Cicatricial," *Dermatol Clin*, 1990, 8(4):701-16 (review).

Baruchin AM, Lustig JP, Nahlieli O, et al, "Burns of the Oral Mucosa: Report of 6 Cases," *J Craniomaxillofac Surg*, 1991, 19(2):94-6.

Halevy S and Shai A, "Lichenoid Drug Eruptions," *J Am Acad Dermatol*, 1993, 29(2 Pt 1):249-55 (review).

Lamey PJ, Rees TD, Binnie WH, et al, "Oral Presentation of Pemphigus Vulgaris and Its Response to Systemic Steroid Therapy," *Oral Surg Oral Med Oral Pathol*, 1992, 74(1):54-7.

Lozada-Nur F, Gorsky M, and Silverman S, Jr, "Oral Erythema Multiforme: Clinical Observations and Treatment of 95 Patients," *Oral Surg Oral Med Oral Pathol*, 1989, 67(1):36-40.

Maron FS, "Mucosal Burn Resulting from Chewable Aspirin: Report of Case," *J Am Dent Assoc*, 1989, 119(2):279-80.

Moncarz V, Ulmansky M, and Lustmann J, "Lichen Planus: Exploring Its Malignant Potential," *J Am Dent Assoc*, 1993, 124(3):102-8.

Mutasim DF, Pelc NJ, and Anhalt GJ, "Cicatricial Pemphigoid," *Dermatol Clin*, 1993, 11(3):499-510 (review).

Rhodus NL and Johnson DK, "The Prevalence of Oral Manifestations of Systemic Lupus Erythematosus," *Quintessence Int*, 1990, 21(6):461-5.

Rogers RS III, Sheridan PJ, and Nightingale SH, "Desquamative Gingivitis: Clinical, Histopathologic, Immunopathologic, and Therapeutic Observations," *J Am Acad Dermatol*, 1982, 7(6):729-35.

Thorn JJ, Holmstrup P, Rindum J, et al, "Course of Various Clinical Forms of Oral Lichen Planus: A Prospective Follow-Up Study of 611 Patients," *J Oral Pathol*, 1988, 17(5):213-8.

Van Dis ML and Vincent SD, "Diagnosis and Management of Autoimmune and Idiopathic Mucosal Diseases," *Dent Clin North Am*, 1992, 36(4):897-917 (review).

Vincent SD, Lilly GE, and Baker KA, "Clinical, Historic, and Therapeutic Features of Cicatricial Pemphigoid: A Literature Review and Open Therapeutic Trial With Corticosteroids," *Oral Surg Oral Med Oral Pathol*, 1993, 76(4):453-9 (review).

PAPILLARY LESIONS

Abbey LM, Page DG, and Sawyer DR, "The Clinical and Histopathologic Features of a Series of 464 Squamous Oral Papillomas," *Oral Surg Oral Med Oral Pathol*, 1980, 49(5):419-28.

Adler-Storthz K, Newland JR, Tessin BA, et al, "Human Papillomavirus Type 2 DNA in Oral Verrucous Carcinoma," *J Oral Pathol*, 1986, 15(9):472-5.

Adler-Storthz K, Newland JR, Tessin BA, et al, "Identification of Human Papillomavirus Types in Oral Verruca Vulgaris," *J Oral Pathol*, 1986, 15(4):230-3.

Budtz-Jorgensen E, "Oral Mucosal Lesions Associated With the Wearing of Removable Dentures," *J Oral Pathol*, 1981, 10(2):65-80 (review).

Harris AM and van Wyk CW, "Heck's Disease (Focal Epithelial Hyperplasia): A Longitudinal Study," *Community Dent Oral Epidemiol*, 1993, 21(2):82-5.

Kamath VV, Varma RR, Gadewar DR, et al, "Oral Verrucous Carcinoma: An Analysis of 37 Cases," *J Craniomaxillofac Surg*, 1989, 17(7):309-14.

Neville B, "The Verruciform Xanthoma: A Review and Report of Eight New Cases," *Am J Dermatopathol*, 1986, 8(3):247-53.

Zunt SL and Tomich CE, "Oral Condyloma Acuminatum," *J Dermatol Surg Oncol*, 1989, 15(6):591-4.

PIGMENTED LESIONS

Bouquot JE and Gundlach KKH, "Odd Tongues: The Prevalence of Common Tongue Lesions in 23,616 White Americans over 35 Years of Age," *Quintessence Int*, 1986, 17(11):719-30.

Brown FH and Houston GD, "Smokers' Melanosis: A Case Report," *J Periodontol*, 1991, 62(8):524-7 (review).

Buchner A and Hansen LS, "Amalgam Pigmentation (Amalgam Tattoo) of the Oral Mucosa: A Clinicopathologic Study of 268 Cases," *Oral Surg Oral Med Oral Pathol*, 1980, 49(2):139-47.

Buchner A, Leider AS, Merrell PW, et al, "Melanocytic Nevi of the Oral Mucosa: A Clinicopathologic Study of 130 Cases from Northern California," *J Oral Pathol Med*, 1990, 19(5):197-201.

Davenport J, Kellerman C, Reiss D, et al, "Addison's Disease," *Am Fam Physician*, 1991, 43(4):1338-42 (review).

Epstein JB and Silverman S, Jr, "Head and Neck Malignancies Associated With HIV Infection," *Oral Surg Oral Med Oral Pathol*, 1992, 73(2):193-200 (review).

Kaugars GE, Heise AP, Riley WT, et al, "Oral Melanotic Macules: A Review of 353 Cases," *Oral Surg Oral Med Oral Pathol*, 1993, 76(1):59-61.

McGarrity TJ, Kulin HE, and Zaino RJ, "Peutz-Jegher's Syndrome," *Am J Gastroenterol*, 2000, 95(3):596-604 (review).

Newland JR and Adler-Storthz K, "Cytomegalovirus in Intraoral Kaposi's Sarcoma," *Oral Surg Oral Med Oral Pathol*, 1989, 67(3):296-300.

Newland JR, Lynch DP, and Ordonez NG, "Intraoral Kaposi's Sarcoma: A Correlated Light Microscopic, Ultrastructural, and Immunohistochemical Study," *Oral Surg Oral Med Oral Path*, 1988, 66(1):48-58.

Rapini RP, Golitz LE, Greer RO, et al, "Primary Malignant Melanoma of the Oral Cavity: A Review of 177 Cases," *Cancer*, 1985, 55(1):1543-51.

Stern SJ and Guillamondegui OM, "Mucosal Melanoma of the Head and Neck," *Head Neck*, 1991, 13(1):22-7.

RED LESIONS

Baughman R, "Median Rhomboid Glossitis: A Developmental Anomaly?" *Oral Surg Oral Med Oral Pathol*, 1971, 31(1):56-65.

Bouquot JE and Gnepp DR, "Epidemiology of Carcinoma *in situ* of the Upper Aerodigestive Tract," *Cancer*, 1988, 61(8):1685-90.

Daley TD and Wysocki GP, "Foreign Body Gingivitis: An Iatrogenic Disease?" *Oral Surg Oral Med Oral Pathol*, 1990, 69(6):708-12.

Espelid M, Bang G, Johannessen AC, et al, "Geographic Stomatitis: Report of 6 Cases," *J Oral Pathol Med*, 1991, 20(9):425-8.

Fisher AA, "Reactions of the Mucous Membrane to Contactants," *Clin Dermatol*, 1987, 5(2):123-36 (review).

Greenberg MS, "Clinical and Histologic Changes of the Oral Mucosa in Pernicious Anemia," *Oral Surg Oral Med Oral Pathol*, 1981, 52(1):38-42.

Kleinman HZ, "Lingual Varicosities," *Oral Surg Oral Med Oral Pathol*, 1967, 23(4):546-8.

Kullaa-Mikkonen A, "Familial Study of Fissured Tongue," *Scand J Dent Res*, 1988, 96(4):366-75.

Massey AC, "Microcytic Anemia. Differential Diagnosis and Management of Iron Deficiency Anemia," *Med Clin North Am*, 1992, 76(3):549-66 (review).

Morimoto K, Kihara A, and Suetsugu T, "Clinico-Pathological Study on Denture Stomatitis," *J Oral Rehabil*, 1987, 14(6):513-22.

Ohman SC, Dahlen G, Moller A, et al, "Angular Cheilitis: A Clinical and Microbial Study," *J Oral Pathol*, 1986, 15(4):213-7.

Shafer WG and Waldron CA, "Erythroplakia of the Oral Cavity," *Cancer*, Shafer WG and Waldron CA, 'Erythroplakia of the Oral Cavity,' Cancer, 1975, 36:1021-8.

Sigal MJ and Mock D, "Symptomatic Benign Migratory Glossitis: Report of Two Cases and Literature Review," *Pediatr Dent*, 1992, 14(6):392-6.

Silverman S, Jr and Lozada F, "An Epilogue to Plasma Cell Gingivostomatitis (Allergic Gingivostomatitis)," *Oral Surg Oral Med Oral Pathol*, 1977, 43(2):211-7.

Van Loon LA, Bos JD, and Davidson CL, "Clinical Evaluation of Fifty-Six Patients Referred With Symptoms Tentatively Related to Allergic Contact Stomatitis," *Oral Surg Oral Med Oral Pathol*, 1992, 74(5):572-5.

SOFT TISSUE ENLARGEMENTS

Barrett AP, "Gingival Lesions in Leukemia: A Classification," *J Periodontol*, 1984, 55(10):585-8.

Bennhoff DF, "Actinomycosis: Diagnostic and Therapeutic Considerations and a Review of 32 Cases," *Laryngoscope*, 1984, 94(9):1198-217 (review).

Buchner A and Hansen LS, "Lymphoepithelial Cysts of the Oral Cavity. A Clinicopathologic Study of Thirty-Eight Cases," *Oral Surg Oral Med Oral Pathol*, 1980, 50(5):441-9.

Butler RT, Kalkwarf KL, and Kaldahl WB, "Drug-Induced Gingival Hyperplasia: Phenytoin, Cyclosporine, and Nifedipine," *J Am Dent Assoc*, 1987, 114(1):56-60.

Cataldo E and Mosadomi A, "Mucoceles of the Oral Mucous Membrane," *Arch Otolaryngol*, 1970, 91(4):360-5.

Chau MN and Radden BG, "A Clinical-Pathological Study of 53 Intraoral Pleomorphic Adenomas," *Int J Oral Maxillofac Surg*, 1989, 18(3):158-62.

Cutright DE, "The Histopathologic Findings in 583 Cases of Epulis Fissuratum," *Oral Surg Oral Med Oral Pathol*, 1974, 37(3):401-11.

de Villiers Slabbert H and Altini M, "Peripheral Odontogenic Fibroma: A Clinicopathologic Study," *Oral Surg Oral Med Oral Pathol*, 1991, 72(1):86-90.

de Visscher JG, "Lipomas and Fibrolipomas of the Oral Cavity," *J Maxillofac Surg*, 1982, 10(3):177-81.

Galloway RH, Gross PD, Thompson SH, et al, "Pathogenesis and Treatment of Ranula: Report of Three Cases," *J Oral Maxillofac Surg*, 1989, 47(3):299-302.

Hirshberg A, Leibovich P, and Buchner A, "Metastases to the Oral Mucosa: Analysis of 157 Cases," *J Oral Pathol Med*, 1993, 22(9):385-90 (review).

Napier SS and Newlands C, "Benign Lympoid Hyperplasia of the Palate: Report of Two Cases and Immunohistochemical Profile," *J Oral Pathol Med*, 1990, 19(5):221-5.

Newland JR, "Benign Lingual Lesions of Intrinsic Origin. Differential Diagnosis," *Postgrad Med*, 1984, 75(4):152-63.

Newland JR, Fasser CE, Smith QW, et al, "Clinical Diagnosis of Localized Intraoral Swellings," *Physician Assistant*, 1983, 7(1):88-99.

Newland JR, Lynch DP, Fasser CE, et al, "Denture-Related Oral Lesions in the Elderly," *Physician Assistant*, 1983, 7(12):37-42.

Nxumalo TN and Shear M, "Gingival Cyst in Adults," *J Oral Pathol Med*, 1992, 21(7):309-13.

Oliver ID and Pickett AB, "Cheilitis Glandularis," *Oral Surg Oral Med Oral Pathol*, 1980, 49(6):526-9.

Patrice SJ, Wiss K, and Mulliken JB, "Pyogenic Granuloma (Lobular Capillary Hemangioma): A Clinicopathologic Study of 178 Cases," *Pediatr Dermatol*, 1991, 8(4):267-76.

Peszkowski MJ and Larsson A, "Extraosseous and Intraosseous Oral Traumatic Neuromas and Their Association With Tooth Extraction," *J Oral Maxillofac Surg*, 1990, 48(9):963-7.

Stal S, Hamilton S, and Spira M, "Hemangiomas, Lymphangiomas, and Vascular Malformations of the Head and Neck," *Otolaryngol Clin North Am*, 1986, 19(4):769-96 (review).

Thomason JM, Seymour RA, and Rice N, "The Prevalence and Severity of Cyclosporin and Nifedipine-Induced Gingival Overgrowth," *J Clin Periodontol*, 1993, 20(1):37-40.

Wright BA and Jackson D, "Neural Tumors of the Oral Cavity. A Review of the Spectrum of Benign and Malignant Oral Tumors of the Oral Cavity and Jaws," *Oral Surg Oral Med Oral Pathol*, 1980, 49(6):509-22 (review).

Zain RB and Fei YJ, "Fibrous Lesions of the Gingiva: A Histopathologic Analysis of 204 Cases," *Oral Surg Oral Med Oral Pathol*, 1990, 70(4):466-70.

SPECIAL TOPICS

"Advisory Statement. Antibiotic Prophylaxis for Dental Patients With Total Joint Replacement. American Dental Association; American Academy of Orthopaedic Surgeons," *J Am Dent Assoc*, 1997, 128(7):1004-8.

American Cancer Society, *Cancer Facts and Figures* 2000, Atlanta, GA.

American Cancer Society, *Cancer Manual*, 8th ed, American Cancer Society, Boston, MA Division, 1990.

Dajani AS, Taubert KA, Wilson W, et al, "Prevention of Bacterial Endocarditis. Recommendations by the American Heart Association," *JAMA*, 1997, 277(22):1794-801.

Durack DT, "Antibiotics for Prevention of Endocarditis During Dentistry: Time to Scale Back?" *Ann Intern Med*, 1998, 129(10):829-31.

Glick M, *Dental Management of Patients With HIV*, Chicago, IL, Quintessence Publishing Co, 1994.

Glick M and Silverman S, "Dental Management of HIV-Infected Patients," *J Am Dent Assoc* (Supplement to Reviewers), 1995.

Glick M, *Clinicians Guide to Treatment of HIV-Infected Patients*, Academy of Oral Medicine, 1996.

Hanssen AD, Osmon DR, and Nelson CL, "Prevention of Deep Periprosthetic Joint Infection," *Instr Course Lect*, 1997, 46:555-67 (review).

Little J, "The American Heart Association's Guidelines for the Prevention of Bacterial Endocarditis: A Critical Review," *Gen Dent*, 1998, 46(5):508-15.

MacPhail LA, Greenspan D, Greenspan JS, et al, "Recurrent Aphthous Ulcers in Association With HIV Infection. Diagnosis and Treatment," *Oral Surg Oral Med Oral Pathol*, 1992, 73(3):283-8.

McCreary C, Bergin C, Pilkington R, et al, "Clinical Parameters Associated With Recalcitrant Oral Candidiasis in HIV Infection. A Preliminary Study," *Int J STD AIDS*, 1995, 6(3):204-7.

National Institutes of Health, Consensus Development Conference on Oral Complications of Cancer Therapies: Diagnosis, Prevention, and Treatment, *J Am Dent Assoc*, 1989, 119(1):179-83 (review).

National Institutes of Health, Consensus Development Conference on Oral Complications of Cancer Therapies: Diagnosis, Prevention, and Treatment, NCI Monograph No. 9, US Public Health Service, Washington, DC, US Government Printing Office, 1990.

Schiodt M, "HIV-Associated Salivary Gland Disease: A Review," *Oral Surg Oral Med Oral Pathol*, 1992, 73(2):164-7.

Ship JA, Grushka M, Lipton JA, et al, "Burning Mouth Syndrome. An Update," *J Am Dent Assoc*, 1995, 126(7):842-53 (review).

Wynn RL, Meiller TF, and Crossley HL, "New Guidelines for the Prevention of Bacterial Endocarditis. American Heart Association," *Gen Dent*, 1997, 45(5):426-8, 430-4.

ULCERATED LESIONS

Bagan JV, Sanchis JM, Milian MA, et al, "Recurrent Aphthous Stomatitis. A Study of the Clinical Characteristics of Lesions in 93 Cases," *J Oral Pathol Med*, 1991, 20(8):395-7.

Balfour HH Jr, Rotbart HA, Feldman S, et al, "Acyclovir Treatment of Varicella in Otherwise Healthy Adolescents. The Collaborative Acyclovir Varicella Study Group," *J Pediatr*, 1992, 120(4 Pt 1):627-33.

Barasch A, Gofa A, Krutchkoff DJ, et al, "Squamous Cell Carcinoma of the Gingiva. A Case Series Analysis," *Oral Surg Oral Med Oral Pathol Oral Radiol Endod*, 1995, 80(2):183-7.

Barnes PF and Barrows SA, "Tuberculosis in the 1990s," *Ann Intern Med*, 1993, 119(5):400-10 (review).

Brannon RB, Fowler CB, and Hartman KS, "Necrotizing Sialometaplasia: A Clinicopathologic Study of Sixty-Nine Cases and Review of the Literature, " *Oral Surg Oral Med Oral Pathol*, 1991, 72(3):317-25 (review).

Choi SY and Kahyo H, "Effect of Cigarette Smoking and Alcohol Consumption in the Aetiology of Cancer of the Oral Cavity, Pharynx and Larynx," *Int J Epidemiol*, 1991, 20(4):878-85.

Hook EW 3rd and Marra CM, "Acquired Syphilis in Adults," *N Engl J Med*, 1992, 326(16):1060-9 (review).

Johnson BD and Engel D, "Acute Necrotizing Ulcerative Gingivitis: A Review of Diagnosis, Etiology and Treatment," *J Periodontol*, 1986, 57(3):141-50 (review).

Mashberg A and Samit AM, "Early Detection, Diagnosis, and Management of Oral and Oropharyngeal Cancer," *CA Cancer J Clin*, 1989, 39(2):67-88 (review).

McKenzie CD and Gobetti JP, "Diagnosis and Treatment of Orofacial Herpes Zoster: Report of Cases," *J Am Dent Assoc*, 1990, 120(6):679-81 (review).

Meiller TF, Kutcher MJ, Overholser CD, et al, "Effect of an Antimicrobial Mouthrinse on Recurrent Aphthous Ulcerations," *Oral Surg Oral Med Oral Pathol*, 1991, 72(4):425-9.

Newland JR, "Oral Ulcers," *Differential Diagnosis II*, Taylor RB (ed), Philadelphia, PA: WB Saunders Co. 1992.

Newland JR, "Oral Ulcers: Keys to Differential and Definitive Diagnosis," *Consultant*, 1989, 29:157-73.

Partridge M and Langdon JD, "Oral Cancer: A Serious and Growing Problem," *Ann R Coll Surg Engl*, 1995, 77(5):321-2.

Patten SF and Tomecki JT, "Wegener's Granulomatosis: Cutaneous and Oral Mucosal Disease," *J Am Acad Dermatol*, 1993, 28:710-8.

Plauth M, Jenss H, and Meyle J, "Oral Manifestations of Crohn's Disease: An Analysis of 79 Cases," *J Clin Gastroenterol*, 1991, 13(1):29-37 (review).

Porter SR and Scully C, "Aphthous Stomatitis - An Overview of Aetiopathogenesis and Management," *Clin Exp Dermatol*, 1991, 16(4):235-43 (review).

Regezi JA, Zarbo RJ, Daniels TE, et al, "Oral Traumatic Granuloma. Characterization of the Cellular Infiltrate," *Oral Surg Oral Med Oral Pathol*, 1993, 75(6):723-7.

Samaranayake LP, "Oral Mycoses in HIV Infection," *Oral Surg Oral Med Oral Pathol*, 1992, 73(2):171-80 (review).

Scully C, "Orofacial Herpes Simplex Virus Infections: Current Concepts in the Epidemiology, Pathogenesis, and Treatment and Disorders in Which the Virus May be Implicated," *Oral Surg Oral Med Oral Pathol*, 1989, 68(6):701-10 (review).

Scully C, "Viruses and Oral Squamous Carcinoma," *Eur J Cancer B Oral Oncol*, 1992, 28B(1):57-9 (review).

Silverman S Jr, "Early Diagnosis of Oral Cancer," *Cancer*, 1988, 62(8 Suppl):1796-9.

Snider DE and Roper WL, "The New Tuberculosis," *N Engl J Med*, 1992, 326(10):703-5.

Spiro RH, "Salivary Neoplasms: Overview of 35-Year Experience with 2,807 Patients," *Head Neck Surg*, 1986, 8(3):177-84.

Spruance SL, Stewart JC, Rowe NH, et al, "Treatment of Recurrent Herpes Simplex Labialis With Oral Acyclovir," *J Infect Dis*, 1990, 161(2):185-90.

Terezhalmy GT, Cottone JA, and Baker BR, "Sexual Diseases Important to Dentistry: Clinical Diagnosis and Treatment," *Dentistry*, 1986, 6(2):7-18.

Vincent SD and Lilly GE, "Clinical, Historic, and Therapeutic Features of Aphthous Stomatitis. Literature Review and Open Clinical Trial Employing Steroids," *Oral Surg Oral Med Oral Pathol*, 1992, 74(1):79-86 (review).

Waldron CA, el-Mofty SK, and Gnepp DR, "Tumors of the Intraoral Minor Salivary Glands: A Demographic and Histologic Study of 426 Cases," *Oral Surg Oral Med Oral Pathol*, 1988, 66(3):323-33 (review).

Wright DG, Dale DC, Fauci AS, et al, "Human Cyclic Neutropenia: Clinical Review and Long-Term Follow-Up of Patients," *Medicine*, 1981, 60(1):1-13.

Wright JM, Rankin KV, and Wilson JW, "Traumatic Granuloma of the Tongue," *Head Neck Surg*, 1983, 5(4):363-6.

WHITE LESIONS

Allen CM, "Diagnosing and Managing Oral Candidiasis," *J Am Dent Assoc*, 1992, 123(1):77-8, 81-2.

Bouquot JE, "Reviewing Oral Leukoplakia-Clinical Concepts for the 1990s," *J Am Dent Assoc*, 1991, 122(7):80-2 (review).

Bouquot JE and Gundlach KKH, "Odd Tongues: The Prevalence of Common Tongue Lesions in 23,616 White Americans Over 35 Years of Age," *Quintessence Int*, 1986, 17(11):719-30.

Boyd AS and Neldner KH, "Lichen Planus," *J Am Acad Dermatol*, 1991, 25(4):593-619 (review).

Durocher RT, Thalman R, and Fiore-Donno G, "Leukoedema of the Oral Mucosa," *J Am Dent Assoc*, 1972, 85(5):1105-9.

Fotos PG, Vincent SD, and Hellstein JW, "Oral Candidiasis: Clinical, Historical and Therapeutic Features of 100 Cases," *Oral Surg Oral Med Oral Pathol*, 1992, 74(1):41-9.

Greenspan D and Greenspan JS, "Significance of Oral Hairy Leukoplakia," *Oral Surg Oral Med Oral Pathol*, 1992, 73(2):151-4 (review).

Holmstrup P and Axell T, "Classification and Clinical Manifestations of Oral Yeast Infections," *Acta Odontol Scand*, 1990, 48(1):57-9 (review).

Jungell P, "Oral Lichen Planus: A Review," *Int J Oral Maxillofac Surg*, 1991, 20(3):129-35 (review).

Kaugars GE, Mehailescu WL, and Gunsolley JC, "Smokeless Tobacco Use and Oral Epithelial Dysplasia," *Cancer*, 1989, 64(7):1527-30.

Marcushamer M, King DL, and McGuff S, "White Sponge Nevus: Case Report," *Pediatr Dent*, 1995, 17(7):458-9.

Mihail RC, "Oral Leukoplakia Caused by Cinnamon Food Allergy," *J Otolaryngol*, 1992, 21(5):366-7.

Moncarz V, Ulmansky M, and Lustmann J, "Lichen Planus: Exploring Its Malignant Potential," *J Am Dent Assoc*, 1993, 124(3):102-8.

Muzyka BC and Glick M, "A Review of Oral Fungal Infections and Appropriate Therapy," *J Am Dent Assoc*, 1995, 126(1):63-72 (review).

O'Grady JF and Reade PC, "*Candida albicans* as a Promoter of Oral Mucosal Neoplasia," *Carcinogenesis*, 1992, 13(5):783-6.

SUGGESTED READINGS *(Continued)*

Picascia DD and Robinson JK, "Actinic Cheilitis: A Review of the Etiology, Differential Diagnosis, and Treatment," *J Am Acad Dermatol*, 1987, 17(2 Pt 1):255-64 (review).

Sciubba JJ, "Oral Leukoplakia," *Crit Rev Oral Bio Med*, 1995, 6(2):147-50 (review).

Sewerin I, "The Sebaceous Glands in the Vermilion of the Lips and Oral Mucosa of Man," *Acta Odontol Scand*, 1975, 33(68 Suppl):13-26.

Silverman S Jr, Gorsky M, and Lozada F, "Oral Leukoplakia and Malignant Transformation: A Follow-Up Study of 257 Patients," *Cancer*, 1984, 53(3):563-8.

Sinor PN, Gupta PC, Murti PR, et al, "A Case-Control Study of Oral Submucous Fibrosis With Special Reference to the Etiologic Role of Areca Nut," *J Oral Pathol Med*, 1990, 19(2):94-8.

van Wyk CW, Staz J, and Farman AG, "The Chewing Lesion of the Cheeks and Lips: Its Features and Prevalence Among a Selected Group of Adolescents," *J Dent*, 1977, 5(3):193-9.

ANATOMIC SITE INDEX

LABIAL MUCOSA - LIP

WHITE LESIONS
Fordyce's Granules 18
Frictional Keratosis 20
Reticular and Plaque-Type Lichen Planus 28
Smoking-Related Leukoplakia 30
Smokeless Tobacco Keratosis 31
Actinic Cheilitis 34

RED LESIONS
Angular Cheilitis 38
Submucosal Hemorrhages 48

ULCERATED LESIONS
Aphthous Ulcers 54
Primary Herpetic Gingivostomatitis 56
Recurrent Herpes 58
Primary Syphilis 62
Ulcers Associated With Systemic Disease 69
Squamous Cell Carcinoma 70

BLISTERING/SLOUGHING LESIONS
Erosive/Bullous Lichen Planus 74
Pemphigus Vulgaris 78
Paraneoplastic Pemphigus 80
Mucosal Burns 81
Erythema Multiforme 82
Lupus Erythematosus 84

PIGMENTED LESIONS
Melanotic Macule 91
Peutz-Jegher's Syndrome 92
Addison's Disease 93

PAPILLARY LESIONS
Verruca Vulgaris 101
Condyloma Acuminatum 103
Focal Epithelial Hyperplasia 104

SOFT TISSUE ENLARGEMENTS
Fibroma 113
Mucocele 115
Hemangioma 120
Cheilitis Glandularis 127

BUCCAL MUCOSA

WHITE LESIONS
Leukoedema 16
White Sponge Nevus 17
Fordyce's Granules 18
Frictional Keratosis 20
Acute Pseudomembranous Candidiasis 22
Chronic Hyperplastic Candidiasis 24
Cinnamon Oil Allergy 26
Reticular and Plaque-Type Lichen Planus 28
Smokeless Tobacco Keratosis 31
Oral Submucous Fibrosis 32

RED LESIONS
Mucosal Allergy 41
Submucosal Hemorrhages 48

ULCERATED LESIONS
Traumatic Ulcer 52
Aphthous Ulcers 54

Secondary Syphilis 63
Ulcers Associated With Systemic Disease 69

BLISTERING/SLOUGHING LESIONS
Erosive/Bullous Lichen Planus 74
Pemphigus Vulgaris 78
Paraneoplastic Pemphigus 80
Mucosal Burns 81
Erythema Multiforme 82
Lupus Erythematosus 84

PIGMENTED LESIONS
Amalgam Tattoo 89
Melanotic Macule 91
Peutz-Jegher's Syndrome 92
Addison's Disease 93
Smoker's Melanosis 94

PAPILLARY LESIONS
Focal Epithelial Hyperplasia 104

SOFT TISSUE ENLARGEMENTS
Pyogenic Granuloma 110
Fibroma 113
Lipoma 119
Hemangioma 120
Neurofibroma 123

GINGIVA

WHITE LESIONS
Frictional Keratosis 20
Cinnamon Oil Allergy 26
Reticular and Plaque-Type Lichen Planus 28
Smokeless Tobacco Keratosis 31

RED LESIONS
Foreign Body Gingivitis 44
Plasma Cell Gingivitis 45

ULCERATED LESIONS
Traumatic Ulcer 52
Primary Herpetic Gingivostomatitis 56
Recurrent Herpes 58
Herpes Zoster 61
Tuberculosis 64
Deep-Seated Fungal Infection/Histoplasmosis 65
Necrotizing Ulcerative Gingivitis 67
Ulcers Associated With Systemic Disease 69
Squamous Cell Carcinoma 70

BLISTERING/SLOUGHING LESIONS
Erosive/Bullous Lichen Planus 74
Cicatricial Pemphigoid 76
Pemphigus Vulgaris 78
Paraneoplastic Pemphigus 80
Erythema Multiforme 82
Lupus Erythematosus 84

PIGMENTED LESIONS
Physiologic Pigmentation 88
Amalgam Tattoo 89
Melanotic Macule 91
Smoker's Melanosis 94
Kaposi's Sarcoma 96
Malignant Melanoma 98

PAPILLARY LESIONS
Verrucous Carcinoma 107

SOFT TISSUE ENLARGEMENTS
Pyogenic Granuloma 110
Peripheral Giant Cell Granuloma 111
Peripheral Ossifying Fibroma 112
Fibroma 113
Epulis Fissuratum 114
Parulis 117
Actinomycosis 118
Gingival Cyst of the Adult 126
Drug-Induced Gingival Hyperplasia 129
Leukemic Gingival Infiltrate 130
Metastatic Carcinoma 131

HARD PALATE

WHITE LESIONS
Frictional Keratosis 20
Acute Pseudomembranous Candidiasis 22
Reticular and Plaque-Type Lichen Planus 28
Nicotinic Stomatitis 33

RED LESIONS
Erythematous Candidiasis 36
Erythroplakia 39
Submucosal Hemorrhages 48

ULCERATED LESIONS
Traumatic Ulcer 52
Primary Herpetic Gingivostomatitis 56
Recurrent Herpes 58
Wegener's Granulomatosis 66
Necrotizing Sialometaplasia 68
Ulcers Associated With Systemic Disease 69
Salivary Gland Carcinoma 71

BLISTERING/SLOUGHING LESIONS
Erosive/Bullous Lichen Planus 74
Pemphigus Vulgaris 78
Mucosal Burns 81
Erythema Multiforme 82
Lupus Erythematosus 84

PIGMENTED LESIONS
Smokers Melanosis 94
Melanocytic Nevus 95
Kaposi's Sarcoma 96
Malignant Melanoma 98

PAPILLARY LESIONS
Squamous Papilloma 100
Verruciform Xanthoma 102
Inflammatory Papillary Hyperplasia 105

SOFT TISSUE ENLARGEMENTS
Benign Salivary Gland Neoplasms 128

TONGUE-DORSAL SURFACE

WHITE LESIONS
White Hairy Tongue 19
Acute Pseudomembranous Candidiasis 22
Reticular and Plaque-Type Lichen Planus 28

RED LESIONS
Stomatitis Areata Migrans 40
Fissured Tongue 42
Atrophic Glossitis 43
Median Rhomboid Glossitis 46

ULCERATED LESIONS
Aphthous Ulcers 54
Primary Herpetic Gingivostomatitis 56
Ulcers Associated With Systemic Disease 69

BLISTERING/SLOUGHING LESIONS
Erosive/Bullous Lichen Planus 74
Pemphigus Vulgaris 78
Paraneoplastic Pemphigus 80
Erythema Multiforme 82

PIGMENTED LESIONS
Black Hairy Tongue 90
Peutz-Jeghers Syndrome 92
Addison's Disease 93

PAPILLARY LESIONS
Verruca Vulgaris 101
Condyloma Acuminatum 103
Focal Epithelial Hyperplasia 104

SOFT TISSUE ENLARGEMENTS
Pyogenic Granuloma 110
Fibroma 113
Hemangioma 120
Lymphangioma 121
Neuroma 122
Neurofibroma 123

TONGUE-LATERAL SURFACE

WHITE LESIONS
Frictional Keratosis 20
Acute Pseudomembranous Candidiasis 22
Chronic Hyperplastic Candidiasis 24
Cinnamon Oil Allergy 26
Reticular and Plaque-Type Lichen Planus 28
Hairy Leukoplakia 29

RED LESIONS
Stomatitis Areata Migrans 40
Submucosal Hemorrhages 48

ULCERATED LESIONS
Traumatic Ulcer 52
Aphthous Ulcers 54
Primary Herpetic Gingivostomatitis 56
Primary Syphilis 62
Tuberculosis 64
Deep-Seated Fungal Infection/Histoplasmosis 65
Ulcers Associated With Systemic Disease 69
Squamous Cell Carcinoma 70

BLISTERING/SLOUGHING LESIONS
Erosive/Bullous Lichen Planus 74
Pemphigus Vulgaris 78
Paraneoplastic Pemphigus 80
Erythema Multiforme 82

PIGMENTED LESIONS
Peutz-Jeghers Syndrome 92
Addison's Disease 93

PAPILLARY LESIONS
Verruca Vulgaris 101
Condyloma Acuminatum 103
Focal Epithelial Hyperplasia 104

SOFT TISSUE ENLARGEMENTS

Pyogenic Granuloma 110
Fibroma 113
Hemangioma. 120
Lymphangioma 121
Neuroma 122
Neurofibroma 123
Lymphoid Hyperplasia 124

TONGUE-VENTRAL SURFACE

WHITE LESIONS

Frictional Keratosis 20
Acute Pseudomembranous Candidiasis. 22
Chronic Hyperplastic Candidiasis 24
Reticular and Plaque-Type Lichen Planus 28

RED LESIONS

Stomatitis Areata Migrans 40
Lingual Varicosities 47
Submucosal Hemorrhages 48

ULCERATED LESIONS

Aphthous Ulcers 54
Primary Herpetic Gingivostomatitis 56
Primary Syphilis 62
Ulcers Associated With Systemic Disease 69
Squamous Cell Carcinoma 70

BLISTERING/SLOUGHING LESIONS

Erosive/Bullous Lichen Planus 74
Pemphigus Vulgaris 78
Paraneoplastic Pemphigus 80
Mucosal Burns 81
Erythema Multiforme 82

PIGMENTED LESIONS

Amalgam Tattoo 89

PAPILLARY LESIONS

Squamous Papilloma 100
Verruca Vulgaris 101
Condyloma Acuminatum. 103
Focal Epithelial Hyperplasia 104

SOFT TISSUE ENLARGEMENTS

Mucocele. 115
Lipoma 119
Hemangioma. 120
Lymphangioma 121
Oral Lymphoepithelial Cyst 125

FLOOR OF THE MOUTH

WHITE LESIONS

Acute Pseudomembranous Candidiasis. 22
Reticular and Plaque-Type Lichen Planus 28
Smoking-Related Leukoplakia 30

RED LESIONS

Erythroplakia 39
Stomatitis Areata Migrans 40
Lingual Varicosities 47
Submucosal Hemorrhages. 48

ULCERATED LESIONS

Aphthous Ulcers 54

Primary Herpetic Gingivostomatitis 56

Ulcers Associated With Systemic Disease 69

Squamous Cell Carcinoma 70

BLISTERING/SLOUGHING LESIONS

Erosive/Bullous Lichen Planus 74

Pemphigus Vulgaris 78

Paraneoplastic Pemphigus 80

Mucosal Burns 81

Erythema Multiforme 82

PIGMENTED LESIONS

Amalgam Tattoo 89

PAPILLARY LESIONS

Proliferative Verrucous Leukoplakia 106

Verrucous Carcinoma 107

SOFT TISSUE ENLARGEMENTS

Ranula 116

Lipoma 119

Oral Lymphoepithelial Cyst 125

SOFT PALATE

WHITE LESIONS

Acute Pseudomembranous Candidiasis 22

Reticular and Plaque-Type Lichen Planus 28

Smoking-Related Leukoplakia 30

RED LESIONS

Erythroplakia 39

Submucosal Hemorrhages 48

ULCERATED LESIONS

Aphthous Ulcers 54

Primary Herpetic Gingivostomatitis 56

Herpangina 60

Secondary Syphilis 63

Ulcers Associated With Systemic Disease 69

Squamous Cell Carcinoma 70

BLISTERING/SLOUGHING LESIONS

Erosive/Bullous Lichen Planus 74

Pemphigus Vulgaris 78

Paraneoplastic Pemphigus 80

Mucosal Burns 81

Erythema Multiforme 82

PAPILLARY LESIONS

Squamous Papilloma 100

Condyloma Acuminatum 103

SOFT TISSUE ENLARGEMENTS

Lymphoid Hyperplasia 124

ALPHABETICAL INDEX

A

Acetaminophen 134
Actinic Cheilosis *see Actinic Cheilitis* 34
Actinic Cheilitis 34
Actinomycosis 118
Acute Pseudomembranous Candidiasis 22
Acyclovir Topical 134
Acyclovir Oral (Capsules or Tablets) 134
Addison's Disease 93
Allergic Contact Stomatitis *see Mucosal Allergy* 41
Allergic Gingivostomatitis *see Plasma Cell Gingivitis* 45
Amalgam Tattoo 89
Amitriptyline 135
Amlexanox 135
Amoxicillin 135
Amoxicillin and Clavulanate Potassium 135
Amphotericin B Cream 3% 136
Amputation Neuroma *see Neuroma* 122
Angular Cheilitis 38
Antibiotic Stomatitis / Sore Mouth *see Erythematous Candidiasis (Acute and Chronic)* 36
Antiseptic Mouth Rinse 136
Aphthous Ulcers 54
Aspirin 136
Atrophic Candidiasis *see Erythematous Candidiasis (Acute and Chronic)* 36
Atrophic Glossitis 43
Attapulgite Suspension 136
Azathioprine 136

B

Bald Tongue *see Atrophic Glossitis* 43
Beefy-Red Tongue *see Atrophic Glossitis* 43
Benign Hyperkeratosis *see Frictional Keratosis* 20
Benign Migratory Glossitis *see Stomatitis Areata Migrans* 40
Benign Mucous Membrane Pemphigoid *see Cicatricial Pemphigoid* 76
Benign Salivary Gland Neoplasms 128
Benzocaine Gel 137
Benzocaine Paste 137
Black Hairy Tongue 90
Blistering / Sloughing Lesions 73
Blood Values, Normal 167

C

Candidal Leukoplakia *see Chronic Hyperplastic Candidiasis* 24
Candidiasis, Acute Pseudomembranous 22
Candidiasis, Atrophic *see Erythematous Candidiasis (Acute and Chronic)* 36
Candidiasis, Chronic Hyperplastic 24
Candidiasis, Erythematous (Acute and Chronic) 36
Canker Sores *see Aphthous Ulcers* 54
Cephalexin 137
Cevimeline 137
Chancre *see Primary Syphilis* 62
Cheilitis Glandularis 127
Chlorhexidine Gluconate 138
Chronic Hyperplastic Candidiasis 24
Cicatricial Pemphigoid 76
Cinnamon Oil Allergy 26
Clarithromycin 138
Clindamycin 138
Clobetasol Propionate Ointment 0.05% 138
Clonazepam 138
Clotrimazole Oral Troche 138

Cold Sores *see Recurrent Herpes* 58
Common Wart *see Verruca Vulgaris* 101
Condyloma Acuminatum 103
Cyclophosphamide 139
Cyclosporine 139

D

Dapsone 139
Deep Fungal Infection / Histoplasmosis 65
Denture Callous *see Frictional Keratosis* 20
Denture Epulis *see Epulis Fissuratum* 114
Denture Stomatitis / Sore Mouth *see Erythematous Candidiasis (Acute and Chronic)* 36
Dexamethasone Elixir 0.5 mL/5 mL 139
Diflunisal 139
Diphenhydramine Liquid (Elixir and Syrup) 140
Docosanol 140
Doxepin 140
Doxycycline Calcium Syrup 140
Doxycycline Hyclate 140
Drug-Induced Gingival Hyperplasia 129
Dry Mouth (Xerostomia) 159

E

Ecchymosis *see Submucosal Hemorrhages* 48
Ectopic Sebaceous Glands *see Fordyce's Granules* 18
Epulis Fissuratum 114
Erosive / Bullous Lichen Planus 74
Erythematous Candidiasis (Acute and Chronic) 36
Erythroleukoplakia *see Erythroplakia* 39
Erythroplakia 39
Erythroplasia *see Erythroplakia* 39
Erythema Migrans *see Stomatitis Areata Migrans* 40
Erythema Multiforme 82

F

Fever Blisters *see Recurrent Herpes* 58
Fibroma 113
Fissured Tongue 42
Fluconazole Tablets 140
Fluocinonide 0.05% (Ointment or Gel) 141
Fluorides 161
Focal Argyrosis *see Amalgam Tattoo* 89
Focal Epithelial Hyperplasia 104
Focal Melanosis *see Melanotic Macule* 91
Fordyce's Granules 18
Foreign Body Gingivitis 44
Foscarnet 141
Frictional Keratosis 20

G

Gabapentin 141
Geographic Tongue *see Stomatitis Areata Migrans* 40
Giant Cell Epulis *see Peripheral Giant Cell Granuloma* 111
Gingival Cyst of the Adult 126
Gingival Hyperplasia, Drug-Induced 129
Gum Boil *see Parulis* 117

H

Hairy Leukoplakia 29
Heck's Disease *see Focal Epithelial Hyperplasia* 104
Hemangioma 120
Hematoma *see Submucosal Hemorrhages* 48
Herpangina 60
Herpes Zoster 61
HIV Infection and AIDS 166

I

Ibuprofen OTC 141
Idiopathic Leukoplakia *see Smoking-Related Leukoplakia* 30
Imiquimod 141
Inflammatory Papillary Hyperplasia 105
Interferon Alfa-2b 142
Iodoquinol and Hydrocortisone 142
Irritation Fibroma *see Fibroma* 113
Itraconazole Capsules 142

K

Kaposi's Sarcoma 96
Ketoconazole Cream 2% 142
Ketoconazole Tablets 142

L

Lactobacillus acidophilus and *Lactobacillus bulgaricus* 143
Leukemic Gingival Infiltrate 130
Leukemic Gingivitis *see Leukemic Gingival Infiltrate* 130
Leukoedema 16
Lichen Planus, Erosive / Bullous 74
Lichen Planus, Reticular and Plaque-Type 28
Lidocaine Viscous 2% 143
Lingual Varicosities 47
Lipoma 119
Lupus Erythematosus 84
Lymphangioma 121
Lymphoid Hyperplasia 124
Lumpy Jaw *see Actinomycosis* 118
Lysine Tablets 143

M

Malignant Melanoma 98
Magnesium Hydroxide / Aluminum Hydroxide Suspension 143
Management of Patients Undergoing Cancer Therapy 156
Median Papillary Atrophy *see Median Rhomboid Glossitis* 46
Median Rhomboid Glossitis 46
Melanocytic Nevus 95
Melanotic Macule 91
Metastatic Carcinoma 131
Methotrexate 143
Methylprednisolone 143
Metronidazole 144
Mucocele 115
Mucosal Allergy 41
Mucosal Burns 81
Mucous Escape Reaction *see Mucocele* 115
Mucous Extravasation Phenomenon *see Mucocele* 115
Mucous Patches *see Secondary Syphilis* 63

N

Naproxen 144
Naproxen Sodium 144
Naproxen Sodium OTC 144
Necrotizing Sialometaplasia 68
Necrotizing Ulcerative Gingivitis 67
Neurofibroma 123
Neuroma 122
Nicotinic Stomatitis 33
Normal Blood Values 167
Nortriptyline 144
NUG *see Necrotizing Ulcerative Gingivitis* 67
Nystatin Oral Suspension 144
Nystatin Topical 144
Nystatin / Triamcinolone Acetate Ointment 145

O

Oral Lymphoepithelial Cyst 125
Oral Submucous Fibrosis 32

P

Palatal Papillomatosis *see Inflammatory Papillary Hyperplasia* 105
Papillary Lesions 99
Paraneoplastic Pemphigus 80
Parulis 117
Pemphigoid, Benign Mucous Membrane *see Cicatricial Pemphigoid* 76
Pemphigoid, Cicatricial 76
Pemphigus Vulgaris 78
Penciclovir Cream 145
Penicillin V Potassium 145
Peripheral Fibroma with Calcifications *see Peripheral Ossifying Fibroma* 112
Peripheral Giant Cell Granuloma 111
Peripheral Ossifying Fibroma 112
Perleche *see Angular Cheilitis* 38
Petechiae *see Submucosal Hemorrhages* 48
Peutz-Jegher's Syndrome 92
Physiologic Pigmentation 88
Pigmented Lesions 87
Pilocarpine Oral 145
Plasma Cell Gingivitis 45
Prednisone 145
Pregnancy Gingivitis *see Pyogenic Granuloma* 110
Pregnancy Tumor *see Pyogenic Granuloma* 110
Preprocedural Antibiotics in Dental Patients 162
Primary Herpetic Gingivostomatitis 56
Primary Syphilis 62
Proliferative Verrucous Leukoplakia 106
Pyogenic Granuloma 110

R

Ranula 116
Recurrent Aphthous Stomatitis *see Aphthous Ulcers* 54
Recurrent Herpes 58
Red Lesions 35
Reticular and Plaque-Type Lichen Planus 28
Ridge Callous *see Frictional Keratosis* 20

S

Salivary Gland Carcinoma 71
Secondary Syphilis 63
Shingles *see Herpes Zoster* 61
Smokeless Tobacco Keratosis 31
Smokers Melanosis 94
Smoker's Palate *see Nicotinic Stomatitis* 33
Smoking-Associated Melanosis *see Smokers Melanosis* 94
Smoking-Related Leukoplakia 30
Snuff Dipper's Cancer *see Verrucous Carcinoma* 107
Soft Tissue Enlargements 109
Speckled Leukoplakia *see Erythroplakia* 39
Squamous Cell Carcinoma 70
Squamous Papilloma 100
Stomatitis Areata Migrans 40
Stomatitis Venenata *see Mucosal Allergy* 41
Submucosal Hemorrhages 48
Suggested Readings 168

T

Tacrolimus 146
Tetracycline Syrup (125 mg/5 mL) 146
Thrush *see Acute Pseudomembranous Candidiasis* 22
Tobacco-Associated Leukoplakia *see Smoking-Related Leukoplakia* 30
Tobacco Pouch Keratosis *see Smokeless Tobacco Keratosis* 31

Traumatic Fibroma *see Fibroma* 113
Traumatic Neuroma *see Neuroma* 122
Traumatic Ulcer 52
Trench Mouth *see Necrotizing Ulcerative Gingivitis* 67
Triamcinolone Acetate in Orabase® 146
Triamcinolone Ointment 146
Tuberculosis 64

U

Ulcerated Lesions 51
Ulcers Associated with Systemic Disease 69

V

Valacyclovir 146
Venereal Wart *see Condyloma Acuminatum* 103
Verruca Vulgaris 101
Verruciform Xanthoma 102
Verrucous Carcinoma 107
Vincent's Infection *see Necrotizing Ulcerative Gingivitis* 67

W

Wegener's Granulomatosis 66
White Hairy Tongue 19
White Lesions 15
White Sponge Nevus 17

Lexi-Comp ONLINE for Dentistry

This powerful Internet-based application provides **real-time** access to all Lexi-Comp dentistry knowledge areas. Simply enter a user name and password on a computer with Internet connectivity and navigate to any content area within three mouse clicks! Drug monographs can be accessed directly from a condition or procedure using built-in links. Detailed photographs and radiographs are included.

- Obtain instant DENTAL ALERTS warning of medications that will influence treatment or cause harmful effects to the patient
    - o Effects on Dental Treatment
    - o Effects on Bleeding
    - o Vasoconstrictor/Local Anesthetic Precautions
    - o Dental Comment
- Easily implement Drug Interaction Analysis into your office workflow
    - o Supplemental Patient Drug Form provided (English/Spanish)
- Compare therapeutic categories to your patient drug regimens to select the most appropriate medication
- Access over 1,000 color photographs and radiographs
- Review nearly 12,000 drugs in the Drug ID module
- Print medication leaflets for your patients in 18 languages
- Utilize Web Search and expand your search capabilities to other qualified health web sites

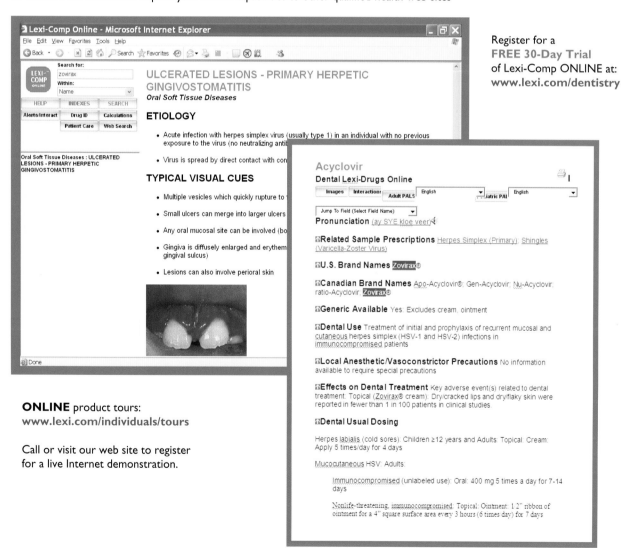

Register for a
FREE 30-Day Trial
of Lexi-Comp ONLINE at:
www.lexi.com/dentistry

ONLINE product tours:
www.lexi.com/individuals/tours

Call or visit our web site to register for a live Internet demonstration.

For more information or to order any of these products, visit our web site or call Customer Service
www.lexi.com/dentistry
1-866-397-3433

Lexi-Comp ON-DESKTOP for Dentistry

Lexi-Comp ON-DESKTOP for Dentistry is the ultimate solution for **Complete Medication Management,** allowing you to store and edit office and patient medication regimens. Our complete library of databases is downloaded to your desktop computer, or hosted on your network server, eliminating the need for a constant Internet connection. Unlimited updates, available during your subscription period, are scheduled to meet your needs and retrieved via the Internet.

Elevate the standard of patient care and help protect your practice from liability with Lexi-Comp ON-DESKTOP for Dentistry.

- ☐ Obtain instant DENTAL ALERTS warning of medications that will influence treatment or cause harmful effects to the patient
    - o Effects on Dental Treatment
    - o Effects on Bleeding
    - o Vasoconstrictor/Local Anesthetic Precautions
    - o Dental Comment
- ☐ Store your office and patient medication lists to help ensure safe treatment plans
- ☐ Easily implement Drug Interaction Analysis into your office workflow
    - o Supplemental Patient Drug Form provided (English/Spanish)
- ☐ Compare therapeutic categories to your patient drug regimens to select the most appropriate medication
- ☐ Access over 1,000 color photographs and radiographs
- ☐ Review nearly 12,000 drugs in the Drug ID module
- ☐ Print medication leaflets for your patients in 18 languages

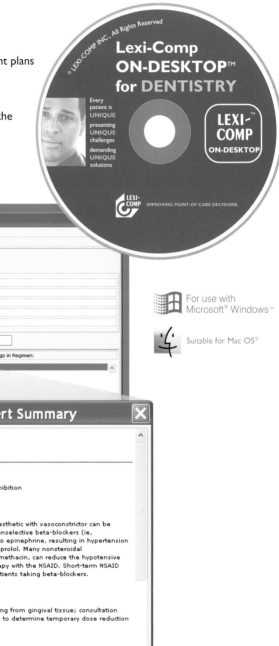

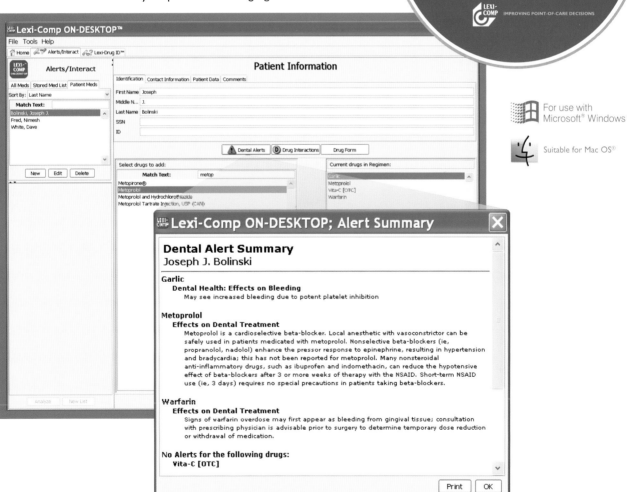

For more information or to order any of these products, visit our web site or call Customer Service

www.lexi.com/dentistry
1-866-397-3433

Lexi-Comp ON-HAND for Dentistry

Lexi-Comp ON-HAND for Dentistry is our top-rated software that provides instant access to point-of-care information on a mobile device. Advanced navigation tools make it easy to find the right information when you need it the most. Updates to our content are available on a daily basis, ensuring you always have the most up-to-date clinical information at your fingertips.

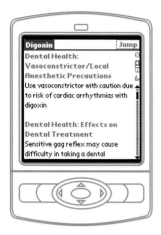

- Dental Lexi-Drugs® includes information on over 7500 drugs
- Up to 30 fields of information including: U.S. Brand Names and Generic Names, Special Alerts, Use, Local Anesthetic/Vasoconstrictor Precautions, Effects on Dental Treatment, Dental Dosing for Selected Drug Classifications, Drug Interactions, Dental Comments, *and more*
- Other available complementary databases include: Lexi-Interact™, Lexi-Natural Products™, Pediatric Lexi-Drugs®, and Stedman's Medical Dictionary for the Health Professions and Nursing

Available on the following platforms:

Drug Information Handbook for Dentistry

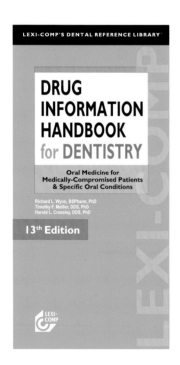

Description

The **Drug Information Handbook for Dentistry**, 13th Edition, is designed for dental professionals seeking information on commonly prescribed medications. Written by dentists, this top-selling reference provides dental-specific content for thousands of medications and the most common herbs and dietary supplements. The user-friendly format lists all medications alphabetically, providing the information you need within seconds —an excellent chair-side reference!

Features

- Contains over 7500 drugs and herbal products, including dental, medical, OTC, Canadian, and Mexican drugs
- Local Anesthetic/Vasoconstrictor Precautions, Effects on Dental Treatment, and Dental Comments
- Drug Interactions, Contraindications, Warnings/Precautions, Common Adverse Effects, Use, Dosage, and Pregnancy Risk Factor

Contents

1) Introduction
2) Alphabetical Listing of Drugs
3) Herbs / Natural Products
4) Medically-Compromised Patients
5) Specific Oral Conditions
6) Sample Prescriptions
7) Appendix
8) Pharmacologic Category Index
9) Alphabetical Index

For more information or to order any of these products, visit our web site or call Customer Service
www.lexi.com/dentistry
1-866-397-3433